Prai...

Vet on the Loose

'This book is just hilarious [and] will no doubt be the first of many in the James Herriot mould.'
Countryman

'It's an engaging account of the situations she encounters where the humans are often more problematic than the animals.'
Irish Independent

'Lively sense of humour, and a pleasant, easy-going writing style. Animal lovers will be well-pleased with her pacy anecdotes.'
Irish Examiner

Vet Among the Pigeons

'Heartwarming ... a very honest portrayal of a demanding job.'
Irish Examiner

'Vet Gillian Hick finds herself challenged in ways the textbooks can't prepare you for!'
Donegal Democrat

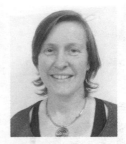

Gillian Hick was born in Dublin and has practised as a vet both in Dublin and in Wicklow. She lives in County Wicklow, where she has her own practice, with her husband, three children and a large assortment of four-legged companions. She has also written *Vet on the Loose* and *Vet Among the Pigeons*.

Vet On
A Mission

Gillian Hick

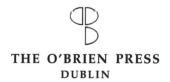

THE O'BRIEN PRESS
DUBLIN

First published 2018 by
The O'Brien Press Ltd,
12 Terenure Road East, Rathgar,
Dublin 6, D06 HD27, Ireland.
Tel: +353 1 4923333; Fax: +353 1 4922777
E-mail: books@obrien.ie; Website: www.obrien.ie
The O'Brien Press is a member of Publishing Ireland.

ISBN: 978-1-78849-026-9

1 3 5 7 9 6 4 2
18 20 22 21 19

Printed and bound by CPI Group (UK) Ltd, Croydon, CR0 4YY.
The paper in this book is produced using pulp from managed forests.

ACKNOWLEDGEMENTS

My thanks, firstly, all to all the readers of *Vet on the Loose* and *Vet Among the Pigeons*, whose kind words and enthusiasm finally made me get *Vet on a Mission* up and running.

Thanks, as always, to all the team at The O'Brien Press, especially to Michael O'Brien for his understanding of my hobby-writer status and to Helen Carr, my editor, for her insight into the world of veterinary medicine!

Many thanks again to Hilary and Joanne from Bridge Street Book shop, our award-winning local bookshop, for all the support throughout the years.

Vet on a Mission is mostly true, with most of the animals (and some of the owners) appearing as themselves. All are based on fact, but a few are amalgams of different cases to protect the identity of the owners! My thanks to all the clients who lent me their animals and, most importantly, to the animals themselves, whose trust — in whatever way they choose to express it! — is always so inspiring. I also credit whatever people-handling skills I have entirely to my animal teachers!

Thankfully, for the writing of this book, I could fall back on the support of the staff of Clover Hill Veterinary Clinic – now that we have grown (above and beyond all expectation) to a level where we have a team to run the practice. Many thanks to Amanda Fitzgerald, Amanda Power, Fiona O'Brien and Roslyn O'Carroll (in the order that they joined the practice) and of course, Striper, the practice cat. Having such a fantastic team allowed me time to write and pursue my many other interests, and generally restore my shredded sanity!

Thanks to John Armstrong, without whose help the practice would probably still be running from a utility room!

Lastly, but most importantly, my thanks to Donal, my husband, and to Molly, Fiona and Jack, my now-teenage children, for their support and inspiration throughout the years.

CONTENTS

CHAPTER 1

THE MISSION

T he sun shone brightly, the air felt fresh and I was bursting with enthusiasm. It was with much regret that I had handed in my notice, some months previously, at Riverside Veterinary Clinic. My time spent in mixed animal practice with Seamus and Arthur had taught me much, but it was time to move on. My eldest daughter Molly was by now at the advanced age of three, her sister Fiona was taking her first steps, and there was a third baby on the way, so I had decided that the rigours of large-animal calls, with a one-in-three night-time rota, was no longer sustainable for the health and wellbeing of my own family, never mind that of my patients! Perhaps if I had known what lay ahead I might have stuck at it for a little longer.

Whether through some pregnancy-hormone-induced neurosis or some strike of divine inspiration, I had decided to open my own veterinary practice. In the early years, I planned to see only small animals so that I would be working from home and then, once the kids were all in the hands of the education system, I would branch back into mixed-animal practice. Donal, my husband, who had his own butcher shop in the historic town of Dalkey, was equally enthusiastic. The plan seemed infallible – until I came head-to-head with the Wicklow County Council planning department.

I had spent many weeks, and even months, of happy hours with an A4 graph pad, drawing and redrawing sketches of my proposed kingdom with Slug, my now ancient but ever faithful pre-child veterinary companion, and instigator of much mischief in my large-animal days, sitting by my side. Then we moved on to the meetings with the architects, consultations with solicitors, letters of recommendation, folders full of planning legislation and notes. The phone calls, the meeting, the draft letters, the engineers' reports, the amended notes. It seemed endless. Finally, Wicklow County Council were happy to suggest that perhaps I should apply for planning for a Methadone clinic as there was clear legislation for such in the constitution but not, they informed me, for a veterinary practice.

Not being one to take no for an answer, I decided to move on. The past week I had spent on the computer, researching rental properties in Wicklow and the surrounding area. Today, I was to meet the three local estate agents to commence plan B.

As Donal usually left around six in the morning to beat the rush hour traffic, my parents duly arrived on the button of nine, packing Molly and Fiona into the back of the car to take them off for some blissful hours of undivided attention.

I quickly checked through my notes before setting off. A list of my basic requirements: ample parking to allow close access for sick or injured animals; a non-residential area to prevent problems with neighbours objecting to barking dogs; ideally a nice area out the back for exercising the patients; soundproof rooms would be a bonus, but not essential; a sufficiently long lease to allow time to get the business up and running. The list went on. Throwing a pen and notebook into my folder, I headed off, brimming with excitement to see where I would start my practice.

The offices of the first estate agent were bright and professional-looking. The middle-aged man listened attentively while I laid out my requirements.

'Yes, I'm getting an idea of the type of property you're looking for,' he started, thoughtfully. 'There might be some difficulties, but I do have one on the books at the moment that might be of interest. If you're free for a while I can get Linda to show it to you.'

I was thrilled to find myself, twenty minutes later, following the car of one of the office staff to view my first property.

'I always wanted to be a vet,' Linda had confided to me as we made our way out to the car park. 'I absolutely love animals!'

The location was perfect. The currently vacant premises was located in the heart of Ashford village, with parking space directly outside and a big glass front that I already envisaged as looking into the waiting room. Once inside, I was slightly disconcerted to see that the layout was totally unsuitable, but the internal walls were flimsy and Linda assured me that change would not be a problem with James, the existing landlord. The lease was for four years and nine months, but he would be happy to have somebody long term. Out the back was a slightly small but well-fenced and homely-looking garden. Already I could clearly see myself sitting out the back, sharing my lunch with the day's in-patients.

In my mind, I could see it happening and could hardly believe that my first day's search might have landed me, if not my dream home, at least a suitable premises for my practice.

Back inside, I pulled out my notebook and started to jot down the internal dimensions. Kneeling down, I carefully pulled up a corner of the carpet to reveal wooden floorboards.

'That might be a bit of a problem,' I said conversationally to Linda. 'We would have to replace the flooring in the whole building.' As I spoke, I was already choosing the colour of the hospital-grade flooring that would compliment the freshly-painted walls, creating a clean yet calming environment for my future patients.

'Oh, I really don't think so,' replied Linda. 'These carpets are in excellent condition – they were only put down two years ago by Martsworth.'

'Yes, it's a shame, but carpets wouldn't be suitable at all for animals. They would be destroyed in no time,' I answered her, surprised that a self-professed animal lover wouldn't see that.

'Oh, but surely you wouldn't have the animals *in* the building with you?' asked Linda, looking shocked. 'Like, wouldn't they all be out in the back garden? I really don't think James would like the idea of animals actually being *in* the building.'

And that was the end of that.

It was almost midday before I made it to the next estate agents and, again, laid out my requirements, this time feeling a little less optimistic. Martin was helpful but doubtful.

'Business is good in the area at the moment,' he told me, 'and rents are high. People want something a little ... well, maybe cleaner, more straightforward, like an office or a shop or something. Your husband is one of the Hicks' butchers, isn't he? I don't suppose he would be interested in a property in the area? We might have a nice unit that would suit him.'

As I made my way up Main Street to the last estate agent, I was beginning to fade. The sun that had shone so brightly as I started my day, shone just a little too brightly now. The weight of my unborn son was starting to bear heavily, and the hill up Wicklow Main Street seemed steeper than usual. I was half tempted to stop somewhere for lunch, but was expecting the girls back home for two so decided to push on. I was starting to feel a little nauseous from the unaccustomed two cups of coffee I had had in my meetings and from the lack of food. Beads of perspiration started to break out on my forehead as I continued up Main Street.

Just on the corner, I spotted two lads selling herrings out

of a fish box, obviously fresh from the morning's catch, and decided to buy a few for a quick lunch back home. It was only after I handed over the ten euro note that I realised I would have to bring them with me into the estate agent's.

The office was hot and at the top of two flights of stairs. I was starting to feel dizzy and could feel my hands shaking as I laid my folder on the table and sank gratefully into the small hard-backed chair, not noticing as the bag slipped out of my hand and the fish slithered gleefully over the (thankfully) tiled floor. Embarrassed, I bent down and eventually gathered all the escapees back into the bag. I definitely felt dizzy as I sat back up and had to wipe the sweat off my brow.

It was only as I pulled out my notebook and started to read out, for the third time, my list of my requirements that I noticed my hands were covered in fish scales, which seemed to have miraculously spread all over my folder, my notebook, the office desk and, I could only assume, my recently mopped brow. Trying to ignore the increasingly fishy smell, I bravely continued though my list.

'So, do you think you might have anything suitable?' I finally enquired, as the estate agent had not uttered a word since the runaway fish episode.

'Do you know,' he began quietly, in a slow, patient voice as though talking to somebody not quite with it, 'my wife has a lovely recipe for herrings. You make a batter with oatmeal and slow roast them in the oven. It's really quite delicious,' he continued kindly. 'Now, why don't you sit there for a few minutes and I'll get one of the girls to make you a nice cup of tea.'

'But what about my rental property?' I replied weakly, clutching on to my folder in one hand and my bag of fish in the other, hoping they would support me through the next dizzy spell.

'Sure I'll be talking to Donal up at the match next weekend, and I can have a chat with him if something comes up.'

By the time Molly and Fiona arrived home, well after the appointed two o'clock, I had abandoned the unfortunate herrings – after all, who knows what they might have caught on the estate agent's floor. I revived myself with a toasted sandwich and was back sitting at the kitchen table, Slug still at my feet, drawing new sketches on yet another A4 graph pad.

CHAPTER 2

DOUBLE JOBBING

Some months later, I found myself lying in bed one night with six-week-old baby Jack lying peacefully in his cradle that his grandad (the original Jack) had handmade when Molly, the eldest, was born. Donal had been temporarily relegated to the relative tranquillity of the spare room. I lay semi-slumbering, one ear tuned attentively towards Jack, except for one small addition, in the form of a forty-kilo Boxer dog lying, attached to a drip, on a veterinary bed on the floor beside me.

My failure to find a suitable premises to rent for the practice, and the lack of time with the imminent arrival of Jack, had led us to alter the plans somewhat. Instead of going for a purpose-built premises, we had decided to convert our eight-foot by-eight-foot utility room into a consulting room that would double as a theatre whenever the need arose. As always, the plans took on a life of their own, and before we knew it a portacabin had been ordered into which we planned to fit second-hand kennels, a few extra sinks and some storage space.

The plan seemed foolproof. Everything was based at home, which would be ideal with three pre-school children. Donal would be home in the evenings, allowing me to run evening clinics, and my mother was on standby to come over one or two mornings a week to be with the kids if I needed to run a morning clinic or had patients in for surgery. As our house was on a one and a half acre site in a quiet rural setting, on what my sister described as a 'rats' motorway', due to the grass growing up the middle of the road, we were unlikely to be overwhelmed with business. When the kids reached school age, I would look again at the option of building or renting a premises or if the clinic wasn't taking off at all, I could simply take a job with one of the local mixed-animal practices.

No matter how many of the hundred and one things we had thought of, there was always the hundred and second that we had overlooked. In the early weeks of the new practice, when it was normal to see one or two animals a day, the Blue Cross had sent me a referral, in the form of an elderly lady with a cat who was apparently in a bad way having been hit by a car. The distraught client followed my directions up the hairpin bends leading to the house, but I had neglected to tell her to come to the back door of the house for the surgery. Instead she arrived, cat draped dramatically across her arms, to the front door. As I was on my own with the kids, I had warned them that I had to treat a sick cat. I planned to admit it for pain relief and stabilisation, knowing that Donal was on the way home at which time I could give it my undivided attention if more intervention was required. With Jack sleeping peacefully in his cradle and Molly and Fiona quietly engrossed in making a 'get well soon' card for the sick cat, I was out the back, setting up a heat lamp in the kennels when the front doorbell rang. I didn't hear the bell from the back of the house, so Molly beat me to the door.

'Are you the lady with the squashed cat? Come on in. Would you like a cup of tea?' she asked her with great enthusiasm all in one breath.

The poor woman looked even more bewildered as I quickly ushered her through to the back room, mentally making a note to put up more signage directing people around to the back door.

Luckily, Ginger the cat was not as traumatised as his owner and all that was needed was some pain relief and instructions for a few days rest (along with a gentle recommendation about neutering in the not-too-distant future).

On the night in question my patient's condition was not so straightforward. George was a stunning Boxer who I had often admired as he strutted around the village, normally accompanied by a gaggle of children. Although great with the kids, he had a reputation of fancying himself as the stud of Glenealy. Numerous other canines had challenged his slot over the years, but with his bulk and attitude of disdain, he had quickly dismissed them all.

However, a bit like David and Goliath of old, George finally met his match in the form a dying wasp late one September evening. He probably never even noticed as he swallowed the striped body, but within minutes his face and tongue started to swell dramatically. His owners found him in the back garden, pacing restlessly with great drools of saliva hanging from his mouth, rubbing his face along the ground to relieve the discomfort. By the time George arrived at the clinic he was very agitated and almost as distressed as his owners, who arrived in their pyjamas as they had been on their way to bed. They were relieved when I suggested that I admit him for the night, even though I expressed my concern at the severity of his reaction.

It might seem bizarre that I could have even considered admitting a severely sick dog with a new baby in the house, and with years of hindsight I myself would be inclined to agree, but at the time, having committed to setting up a practice and by accepting clients, I was automatically obliged to provide a twenty-four/seven emergency service for all registered patients. Unlike the GPs who can roll over in bed and send their patients by ambulance to the nearest A and E hospital, in the case of vets, the GP provides the A and E service too! George was a registered patient of mine, so I was obliged to treat him.

Of course there were other vets in the area, but they too had to provide their own cover (although they all had more than one vet, and so could share the nights). Although some practices shared the rota, I was most certainly not in a position to be providing cover for other busier practices, where I would have to go out on large-animal calls so that effectively left me on my own providing twenty-four/seven cover.

Quite apart from the legalities of it all, with the state George was in, there was no way I could do anything other than admit him, as I watched him gasping for breath, tongue hanging out and eyes beginning to bulge with the sheer effort of drawing breath.

Anyway, George the Boxer was not remotely interested in veterinary standards as he slumbered noisily by my bed-side that night. Slug was probably more put out than any of us, as she had been relegated from her usual bed to the kitchen for the night. Her early years of being used for dog-fighting before I 'kidnapped' her, meant that she couldn't be totally trusted with other dogs although she was now in her mid-teens and clearly at a stage in her life that she was preparing for her departure.

Before long, the mixture of intravenous steroid, an antihistamine and a mild sedative to relax him seemed to be working effectively for George. A snoring Boxer is one thing, but a Boxer with a combination of a more than usually restricted airway and a sedative is another thing altogether. Each time Jack woke to feed, which he did regularly that night, he was highly entertained by the sputtering and snorting at the other side of the bed and giggled loudly every time a particularly explosive snore erupted. At one stage, the snoring became so violent that I was concerned that I would have to fully anaesthetise and intubate George if he didn't improve. This was causing me anxiety, as George had first come to me only a few weeks previously and his owner was concerned about a seizure he had had a few weeks earlier. Although he recovered uneventfully, when she heard of the new practice opening, she decided it was a good opportunity to get him checked. At the time, I had advised her that epilepsy was not uncommon in his breed and that if they became any more frequent we would do further investigation and perhaps consider medicating him.

Apart from now realising that it was almost four in the morning as I gazed bleary-eyed at the alarm clock, I really was not keen to anaesthetise him unless absolutely necessary. Thankfully, I remembered that one of my college friends, who was working in an emergency centre on the other side of the world, would be the ideal phone-a-friend as four in the morning in Ireland would equate with her normal working day.

She picked up the phone on the first ring and was thrilled to hear from me as we hadn't spoken since Jack's arrival.

She was not so thrilled when she heard why I was ringing her.

'What are you thinking of? Have you not enough to be doing? Why didn't you just tell them to ...?'

Well, I won't finish her most uncaring approach to a patient in distress.

Grudgingly, she consulted with their on-site anaesthetist,

while I wondered how two people with the same degree could end up in two such drastically different jobs and practices. She came back with a few suggestions for medications, nothing that changed the way I was treating George, but it was nice to have the reassurance (even though she did end the conversation by telling me that talking to me was the best form of contraception she had ever come across!)

Within minutes of the call, George took a few extra-deep snorts, let off a few good blasts or air of the variety available in copious amounts and known only to owners of Boxers, and then miraculously seemed to settle. By early morning he was well enough to move back into the kennels, and seemed disappointed that I wasn't in form for some play. The owners were delighted when I rang them to fill them in on (an edited version of) the night's events.

They arrived to collect him some time later, still in their pyjamas, although I by now was well up and dressed, ably assisted by Molly and Fiona, who had a slight tussle over picking Jack's outfit for the day. I was too exhausted to do up the bill, as I couldn't get my head around thinking up a fair price for intensive night care, but they promised to call up the next day to settle up.

As the practice was still in its infancy, I only had to deal with a few phone calls until the evening clinic by which stage Donal was back home to mind the kids. Although the girls were in their usual high spirits, Jack slept more that day, clearly worn out from giggling at the snoring, farting Boxer during the night! We spent most of the day on the couch in relative peace, although I did get a chance to do up the bill for George's owners in the afternoon.

As it turned I needn't have bothered as they never did come up the next day to pay, nor the week after, nor at the end of the month when I sent another bill, nor the month after that again. After the third month, when my bill was returned with an 'owner has moved – no forwarding address' stamp from the local post office, I realised that anaesthetic regimes for toxic epileptic Boxers was not the only aspect to running a business that I had to get to grips with!

CHAPTER 3

THE DOG LADY

I don't know why, but I clearly remember the first phone call I ever received from Eve Wilson. Perhaps it was the fact that she had one of those very soft, gentle voices that instantly invited you to slow down and listen. She was enquiring about getting her female spaniel neutered as she was in heat and although Eve had bred from her in the past, she wasn't planning on it again. I agreed that neutering would be the best option, but advised that it would be best to wait until she was out of heat.

Eve agreed immediately, saying, 'I'll be guided by whatever you think is best.'

I took her details and told her I would keep a note on her file and contact her in three months' time as this would be the safest time for Juno the spaniel.

She seemed surprisingly grateful, in a quiet way.

I didn't think any more of it until the following week when she rang again, this time to make an appointment for another dog.

By now, I had become accustomed to clients filling me in with their entire schedule for the week as they tried to fit in an appointment, usually requiring me to reorganise mine. This was never the case with Eve, and she always graciously accepted the first appointment I offered her, so later that evening, I became acquainted with Freddie, a scruffy terrier type.

Often when you form an opinion of someone in your mind, when you meet them they don't look anything like you imagined. In Eve's case, it was as though I had actually met her before. Although there were a few new clients that evening, as soon as Eve stepped out of the old clapped-out Ford Cortina, it was as though I recognised her or had known her for years. She was exactly as I had pictured her – a petite woman, almost frail-looking and yet with an inner strength. Her hair was silvery-grey and shoulder length, carelessly tied up in a simple rubber band. Her eyes were grey-blue, and when she reached out to shake my hand we held each other's gaze and for a moment I again felt as though we had previously met.

Freddie had always had an ongoing itchy tummy, but the rash had flared up in recent days. His skin was warm to the touch and his hind-limb reflexively began to scratch as I ran my hands gently along his body. As I questioned Eve about his history she listened attentively and filled me in on his diet, his sleeping area, his anti-parasite treatment and other matters, which would give me some clues as to his recent flare-up. I explained to Eve that chronic skin cases could be very difficult to resolve completely, but that I was hopeful that by changing him from his current straw bedding and applying some mild steroid cream, it should settle down.

'Do you think it was the straw that set him off?' she questioned anxiously. 'He's one of my outdoor dogs, and the neighbouring farmer offered me a few broken bales last week. It's such a pity; they looked so nice and snug on the fresh bed,' she trailed off as much to herself as to me.

'Do you have many other dogs?' I asked her, assuming as she had mentioned that Freddie was an outdoor dog, that she had indoor dogs too.

In an instant, it was as though I had erected a steel barrier between us. The gentle, open demeanour suddenly disappeared and Eve quickly offered to settle her account out of a small plastic bag consisting of a few well-folded notes in addition to a mix of coins. Then she was gone.

The queue of cars around the back of the house left me no time to wonder how I had offended her, but it was not long before I saw her again. This time with a small black dog.

Mrs Black, as she was aptly called, was a very pretty, dainty spaniel type, whose ears were so long that the hair actually touched the ground as she walked. However, unlike Freddie who spent the entire duration of his consultation enthusiastically trying to lick me and climb up into my arms, Mrs Black seemed terrified. She clung frantically to Eve when she lifted her to put her on the table, and as soon as I laid my hands on her, her whole body began to quiver.

Although Eve showed none of the resistance from our previous conversation, her face tightened up into a frown as she explained that Mrs Black had had a bad experience in another veterinary practice. Although I didn't encourage her to expand on it, I did suddenly realise that I had never even asked her who her previous vet had been. As a policy, I would never see another vet's patient without first asking the vet's permission and getting an-up-to-date history for the animal. This is both as a professional courtesy to my colleagues and also in the best interest of my patient. Clearly, Eve had at least three dogs that I knew of, so she must have been to another vet before now.

'I'll be coming to you from now on,' she told me when I questioned her. 'None of them are being treated for anything, so you need have no worries.'

The discussion was clearly closed.

Although I wasn't entirely happy with the situation, I was reluctant to push it as I didn't want to encourage a discussion on why she was unhappy with her previous vet. Although under normal circumstances I would have been suspicious, as often clients want to change vets claiming to have been badly treated when they actually owe a lot of money to a previous vet. In Eve's case, although she clearly was not flush with money, there was something about her that I warmed to. I could sense that she was an innately private person, and yet I completely trusted her.

Examining Mrs Black was not easy as she was so tense. As I had never met her before, I didn't know if the tension was just from fear or a part of her medical condition. I took my time with her, encouraging her to relax. It appeared that not only had she severe neck pain, but all her back muscles were in spasm too. Despite my best efforts, I wasn't able to carry out any form of useful neurological exam as she clung to Eve for the entire duration of the consultation. When, at my request, Eve placed her gently on the floor, Mrs Black refused to move and stood in under the consulting table with her neck bent down so far that her nose was almost touching the floor.

'Let me take her this time,' I said. I gently picked my reluctant patient up and, although she bared her teeth at me, she never budged otherwise.

'It's most likely some sort of muscle spasm, but I can't rule out other neurological or spinal causes as she is so nervous,' I told Eve as I gently placed Mrs Black back in her arms.

'Yes, I thought it could be a disc, or I was even afraid she might have broken a bone in her neck. I don't see how she could have done it, because she sleeps in my bed with me and she just woke up like this.'

It's always difficult in veterinary trying to work out what is the best option for both patient and client. While I wasn't really happy with the idea of sending Mrs Black home with anti-inflammatories and instructions for cage rest, I didn't feel from my dealings with Eve so far that sending her to the veterinary referral hospital was going to be an option.

'Why don't I give her a strong painkiller now to make her comfortable, and then I'll give you some anti-inflammatories for her for the next few days. I'm sure that she'll be happier going home with you than if I kept her in, but keep her totally confined and then then let me know how she's doing in the morning,' I suggested.

'Oh, thank God,' replied Eve, 'I thought you were going to say that she would need an x-ray, and I really don't have the money for that at the moment.'

Realistically, I knew that if Mrs Black didn't respond to conservative treatment, she would need much more than just a simple radiograph, but I decided against stressing Eve any further at that moment.

'Let's just see how she gets on tonight. Ring me in the morning or at any stage if she gets any worse,' I replied, opening the door for her to take the still-quivering Mrs Black back to the car.

🐾 🐾 🐾

Eve did ring early the next morning to say that Mrs Black was significantly improved.

'She's eating now, and when I carried her out to the toilet she was moving more comfortably.'

Over the next few days Eve rang me daily to update me on the slow but positive progress of Mrs Black. I was impressed by her attention to detail and her diligence in carrying out my instructions exactly as prescribed, as Eve, to me, looked like someone who could do with looking after herself. On the few occasions we had met, despite her strong personality, she seemed terribly frail. I wondered vaguely about her history as she had casually mentioned on one occasion that she lived alone. She was clearly smart and well educated, but other than that, I knew nothing about her.

'Maybe I should bring her up to you to let you check her,' she suggested at the next phone call.

'If you can, that would be great,' I replied, eager to check up on the little dog. I had been reluctant to suggest it as Eve lived quite some distance away and I was conscious of not putting her under pressure. I had found that in the short time I had known her, I looked forward to her calm and gentle personality and welcomed our brief interludes in the madness of daily life.

It was almost dark that evening by the time the clinic started. I had to wait until the end to see Mrs Black, as Eve insisted on letting everyone else go before her. I couldn't help wondering if she didn't have much to go home to. Mrs Black had improved dramatically and I was able to manipulate her neck through a full range of motion, although she quivered dramatically throughout. Once I was happy with her, I gently placed the little spaniel back down on the floor, thinking she would feel less anxious as we discussed her aftercare in terms of gradually reintroducing her exercise.

'Let me just go out to the car and get her lead,' said Eve, opening the consulting room door. In a flash, Mrs Black, who had been huddled nervously under the table, shot out and disappeared into the darkness. Although upset by the little dog's apparent terror, I was not overly concerned for her safety as I knew that the small area around the house was fully fenced. It still took us some time to catch Mrs Black – we pursued the little black shadow in circles around the house before she finally came to rest under a bush. I backed off, allowing Eve to gently pull her out to safety. With Mrs Black securely back in the car, Eve seemed almost to evaporate.

Although she was one of those seemingly ageless people, as she leaned over the surgery table, her previously clear skin appeared drawn and her lips had a slight blueish tinge. Her breathing, I noticed with alarm, had become audibly laboured. Quickly pulling a chair from the next room, I sat her down.

'My handbag,' she gasped, pointing feebly to her bag, which was lying in the corner.

I placed the bag in her lap and watched as she fumbled in it before pulling out two inhalers. I supported her as she haltingly drew from them and sat quietly by her side, her hand gently resting in mine. Over the next few minutes she gradually relaxed and her colour returned to near normal, although she was still pale. My head was screaming at me to call an ambulance, but I felt that this would have upset Eve even more.

'Please let me drive you home, Eve,' I asked, knowing that Donal was in for the evening with the kids. As I expected, she adamantly refused, and only after much persuasion agreed to have a cup of tea before she left. Under no circumstance could I cajole her into the kitchen, so we sat side by side in the consulting room sipping at the hot sugary tea, although she wouldn't so much as look at the plate of biscuits. I felt greedy as I devoured a handful, not having eating since much earlier that day.

As she recovered, Eve began haltingly to tell me just a little about herself; how her mother used to breed show dogs and she had grown up with them. She had never left home, and continued living there after her parents had died.

'I gave up breeding once my mother died,' she told me, a little sadly, I felt. 'It wasn't so easy to get really good homes for the dogs and I just hated letting them go. Then people started to bring me dogs that others couldn't look after. It can be a little tight sometimes with so many to feed.'

I sat quietly and listened to her story being very careful not to question her as I was aware of her strong sense of privacy.

When the tea was finished, Eve seemed to come fully back to herself, but as she left she took my hand and thanked me. 'I'm so sorry to have troubled you,' she said, 'but thank you so much for listening to the rambling of an old lady.'

'It's lovely to have a chat,' I assured her. 'And if there is ever anything I can do to help, please do just ask. Or,' I added, 'if you ever want me to call out to you if you're not feeling well, it's no bother at all.'

Eve insisted on paying her bill, and then she was off, Mrs Black sitting patiently on the passenger seat beside her.

I rang Eve the next morning ostensibly to check on Mrs Black, but really to reassure myself that Eve had got home safely. She sounded in good spirits so when I didn't hear from her over the next few weeks I assumed that all was well with both herself and Mrs Black.

It was late one evening when I got a phone call from a lady who told me that we had met briefly in the clinic once with her mother's elderly cat.

She went on to assure me that both her mother and elderly cat were doing fine, so I wondered why she was ringing me late on a Friday night. But when she told me that her mother lived next door to Eve Wilson, I was immediately concerned.

'I saw your business card on Eve's fridge when I was in this morning and thought I should let you know that she passed away last night.'

The instant she told me, I felt like I had always known this was going to happen. It turned out that Eve's intense sense of privacy had ensured that nobody knew that her frailty was due to a serious underlying illness – one for which she had refused any but the most basic medical intervention, preferring instead to stay with her beloved dogs. Eve had passed quietly in her own home with her beloved companions.

Although initially I felt overwhelmed with grief that the gentle lady had so little trust in the world that she could not have asked for help, I finally accepted that this was the way she had wanted it. All I could do now was to help organise things for her loyal companions; I and others did this over the following days and weeks. Ironically, Mrs Black, the only one of her dogs who had been terrified of me, ended up coming to live with us as, whether due to the stress of the change in her circumstance or not, her symptoms flared up again, so that I had to take her home with me.

And on the very day of Eve's passing, Slug, our beloved first child – as Molly had informed the local health nurse – decided that her time had come. Although I was the one who had depressed the plunger of the lethal injection as she took her last breath, she had decided herself that morning as she stared unknowingly at me, unable to lift her once-feisty head from the bed. In a funny way, when I heard that Eve had passed, I was glad that they went together, knowing that two such precious souls would surely find each other.

If Slug had still been with us, I wouldn't have dared to

introduce Mrs Black into the house, but with that gaping empty space in the kitchen, it seemed the right thing to do. Although she had no experience of children that I knew of, she seemed particularly drawn to Molly and Fiona, and would happily spend hours lying under Jack's cot as he slept. Mrs Black ended up living to an old age, exactly how long I'm not sure, as I never knew her age when she came to us, but certainly well into her late teens if not beyond. In a funny way, the little spaniel was remarkably similar in temperament to Eve – a very quiet presence in the house, but with her own ways of doing things. I felt that Eve would have approved of her choice of new home.

CHAPTER 4

A MIRACULOUS ESCAPE

At times, veterinary is a strange career – even without running a business from a utility room with the help and assistance of three small children. Many people complain about the monotony of their job; the life of a vet can also be monotonous, but there are moments when I feel slightly envious of those who are reasonably confident in the morning that they know what they will be doing in the afternoon. In veterinary, a simple phone call can drastically alter the day's best laid plans.

On the day in question, the morning clinic had run smoothly, and I quickly tended to my two in-patients. Cheeky, a miniature Jack Russell, had heroically allowed me to bathe and trim back an infected ingrown toenail without complaint, while Rusty, an enormous oversized chocolate Labrador, had dissolved into a quivering mess as soon as I approached his inflamed ear. In the end, I had to sedate him before being able to thoroughly flush the ear canal which, judging by the amount of sticky black discharge, had been infected for some time. Taking a final examination with the otoscope to satisfy myself that the job was complete, I was just picking up his chart to write up his medications for discharge when the phone rang.

With one hand on Rusty's lead, I picked up the phone with the other and could hear several voices and shouting in the background. By the time Martin, the client, spoke, I knew my quiet lunch before collecting the kids was a thing of the past. Apparently Spud, an over-inquisitive yard collie, had been busy investigating a suspected rat among the bales of silage while her owner was out feeding their cattle. Just as Martin had directed the spike on the tractor into the pit to lift a bale, Spud had spotted the errant rat and dived in between the bales of silage. With the most astounding ill-timing, the spike of the tractor had completely impaled Spud, going right through from one side of her belly and appearing out the other. I can only imagine how the owner felt, looking at his much-loved yard collie lying totally motionless as Martin and his son struggled to pull her off the large metal spike.

'She's lying in the straw, but she looks like she doesn't know we're here,' gasped Martin over the phone. 'I think she's done for.'

'Just wrap her carefully in something warm and bring her straight in,' I told him, anxious not to waste any more time with a dog that was clearly going into shock and would most likely be dead on arrival.

In the twenty minutes it took them to arrive, I quickly set up the anaesthetic machine, heated fluids and prepared for abdominal surgery, but all the while I was thinking that my efforts were probably going to be wasted. It was more likely that Spud would be dead by the time she got here, from some form of massive internal haemorrhage or ruptured organs.

I stood quietly checking that everything was ready to have the luckless Spud anaesthetised and out of pain as soon as possible whatever the outcome. Only when everything was in place did I allow myself to think back to a previous similar case – probably one of the most traumatic I ever dealt with back in my early days as a new graduate, which often came back to haunt me.

※ ※ ※

I had been doing a locum job for a week in an inner-city branch practice when a call had come from the guards. Would I be able to carry out a post-mortem on a dead dog? I was surprised, as the guards usually did not take much interest in domestic pets.

When the young guard, looking fresh out of college, arrived at the surgery, he filled me in on the background to the case. Two families had been involved in an ongoing feud, during which a man had been beaten and left tied up in a deserted woodland. He eventually managed to escape, but in retaliation, some of his family members had stolen the other family's dog and impaled it on the metal spikes of a local graveyard. The dog had been found the next morning, frozen solid on the spike as the incident had occurred in the depths of winter. The fire brigade had been called and the firemen had cut the spikes from the railing; the dog was delivered to us in the surgery complete with two roughly cut metal bars piercing her mutilated body.

Although I never knew the dog, and never saw her when she was alive, her case had a greater impact on me than many others that had come and gone, been treated and forgotten about. For the duration of the lengthy post-mortem examination, which I carried out the next day when the body had finally thawed, I felt numb, unable to even think how the poor animal must have felt or suffered before she died. The only consolation was that with the extent of her injuries I felt sure her death must have been quick.

Equally, my mind dwelled on the perpetrators. What sort of people must they have been? How could any normal, sane person even begin to think up such an idea, never mind carry it out? How had they felt, or what were they thinking, as they hoisted the considerably sized dog up over the railing? Had they watched until the dog died? Had they laughed? Had they cried? Had they felt any sense of remorse? Any sense of uneasiness? Were they even aware that something had gone horribly wrong with their lives?

The guards had only given me scant details as to the background as there were multiple court cases pending. I knew that there were appalling injustices on both sides, but nothing could justify the wanton and savage abuse of this innocent dog.

Although I never met the people that carried out the act – and once my report had been submitted, I never heard any more details about the outcome of the case – I never forgot about them. Over the years, my initial anger towards the people subsided and – maybe with time or maturity or life experience – I have come to have sympathy for them. I still think about them. Who knows if they are still alive? They too could have become victims of drug abuse or violence. They could be serving multiple prison sentences or they could have committed suicide. I can't believe that, unless they were lucky enough to have had some sort of major intervention, they themselves could be in a happy place having carried out and witnessed such a terrible deed. Even if society had forgiven them, how could they ever forgive themselves?

As I stood waiting, the familiar waves of nausea washed over me, as they always do while thinking back to that post-mortem. The skidding of car tyres interrupted my reverie and in an instant I pushed away all thoughts of Tilly, as I named her myself.

Spud was lying on a duvet in the back of the jeep. Her entire body quivered as I gently laid my hands on her. Her eyes were constricted and focused on a faraway point in the manner of a dog that is in major shock. Quickly checking her gums, I was surprised to see that her colour, although pale, was not totally blanched. Martin, the owner was, if anything, in a worse state than his dog.

'It might not be unreasonable to just put her to sleep. The chances of her pulling through this are very poor,' I explained, justifying it as much to myself as to the owner.

Although he was a big man, Martin's reply came out in a whisper.

'Just do anything you can if you can save her, but don't let her suffer anymore.' His whisper was barely audible over the intermittent moans emanating from Spud.

I was happy to hear those words. This gave me permission to immediately anaesthetise Spud, despite the fact that it may not be safe to do so, considering her shock level. Once asleep, Spud would feel no more pain and then I could go in surgically to examine the extent of the damage. If the damage was irreparable, we could simply change the fluid in the giving set from the heated saline to an overdose of anaesthetic, which would allow her to drift off into oblivion.

I did feel sorry sending Martin away so quickly in his state of shock, but I knew the best thing I could do for him was to take care of Spud.

Within minutes, Spud's ordeal was over and she lay peacefully on the operating table oblivious, to the drama that had been unfolding over the previous half hour. As she slept, I clipped and prepared the surgical site to allow access not only to the two puncture wounds, but to her entire abdomen, in case I needed to explore further. The penetration wound on the right-hand side was dangerously close to her rib cage. The exit wound on the far side was smaller, but at an angle indicating the spike had passed diagonally through her body, putting all her vital abdominal organs at risk. Ignoring the actual penetration wound, I made a large incision through her midline, allowing me access to her entire abdomen.

As I extended the incision, I realised that I was holding my breath thinking back to the devastation I had found and painstakingly recorded in Tilly's abdomen – how the large amount of clotted blood had floated freely in the abdomen, how the stomach had been ripped open, allowing the digestive contents to spill freely, mixing with the clotted blood. The guard that had come to observe the post mortem and take notes of my findings had excused himself long before I got to the point where I discovered that the vascular attachment of the spleen had been severed by the blunt force of the spike and the second spike had penetrated between the muscle of the two adjacent ribs, causing a large hole in the rib cage and a punctured lung. I could hear the guard heaving outside and he was ashen faced when he returned apologetically some time later.

Gently, I allowed myself to take a few breaths, trying to focus on Spud, who still had some chance of being helped, observing how my hand was still slightly shaking as I continued the lengthy incision. To my relief, on this occasion, there was no obvious free blood in the abdomen, no stomach contents, nor anything else. In fact, if I had not known otherwise, the abdomen, on initial examination, looked remarkably normal. Usually, exploratory laparotomies are carried out when investigating animals with a foreign body blocking the gut, or investigating cancerous mass, or other equally sinister situations. So it was pleasant not to be greeted with the smell of infected peritoneal fluids or a purple and rank necrotic piece of intestine.

Initially, I carried out a general examination and then, as there was nothing abnormal obviously visible, I began to carry out a more carefully systematic examination of each organ. Thankfully, the first point of penetration was just in front of the diaphragm, the large muscle that separates the heart and lungs in the thorax from the other organs like the liver and kidneys and stomach and intestines in the abdomen.

The liver showed absolutely no signs of damage as the large blunt spike had obviously bounced off the edge and passed uneventfully by the stomach. Carefully I checked both right and left kidneys. The spleen was exactly where it should have been – the large vessels pulsing away happily unaware of how close the point of the spike must have passed by. The intestines looked perfectly normal, as their loose attachments had clearly allowed the spike to pass through as they spilled around the edges. The bladder was intact. Throughout, I could feel Spud's rhythmic, relaxed

breathing as she inhaled a mixture of oxygen and anaesthetic gas.

'This is really weird,' I finally spoke out loud. 'Everything
looks absolutely normal.'

Another thorough examination confirmed that everything was exactly where it should be. Apart from the two
lacerations where the spike had penetrated both sides of the
abdominal wall, Spud had escaped miraculously unharmed.
Mindful of the many millions, if not billions of trillions,
of bacteria that might have gained entry on the spike as
it passed through her abdomen, I set about lavaging the
entire cavity by flushing some four litres of sterile saline
through to reduce the risk of Spud developing peritonitis.
After the third litre, one small wisp of silage did emerge
from between two pieces of intestine. I was almost grateful
for the evidence as the whole surgery was beginning to feel
a little surreal.

The second laceration was relatively easy to repair, but the
first took a bit more attention and effort, as the spike had penetrated high up on the body wall, making it difficult to get
decent access to close the various muscle layers. By the time I
had placed the final suture in the large abdominal incision over
an hour had passed.

Spud recovered uneventfully in the kennels, wrapped in a
heated blanket and with a heat lamp. As I monitored her over
the remainder of the day and the next morning she seemed

comfortable without needing the heavy-dose pain relief that I had prepared just in case. Her temperature remained stable the next day, indicating that the thorough lavage of her abdomen had done its job.

When Martin came to collect her the following morning she trotted out the door and jumped into the back of the jeep as though nothing had happened. I suspect that it took Martin a lot longer to recover!

CHAPTER 5

SCHOOL TALKS

It was with a sense of trepidation that I awoke that morning. Before I was fully conscious, my mind started to scan through the possible reasons for this feeling of unease. Had I a particularly complex surgical case pending? Perhaps a difficult owner due in with a tricky case? Was the clinic double-booked from 8.30 this morning? Had one of the kids a potentially serious medical appointment pending?

No. Suddenly it came to me in a rush. Today was the day of the dreaded school talk.

A very noble and worthwhile initiative had been set up by Veterinary Ireland some years previously, whereby vets were invited to make themselves available to local primary schools and other community-based organisations for the purpose of giving talks. The thought of having the opportunity to enlighten the next generation to the joys and responsibilities of pet ownership seemed too good to miss, so I enthusiastically put my name forward. In my early days I had been through a harrowing experience of giving a talk to over two hundred inner-city Dublin secondary school kids, but I figured that the small class numbers in rural schools and the general innocence of pre-teens would be well within my capabilities.

For the first year, I had carefully planned my talk and even gone so far as write out notes, which I then converted to prompt sheets before each session. I had carefully thought out how to deal with various issues, such as neutering and spaying, for the younger and older groups, having been exposed to some valuable in-house training by Molly on this very issue.

Although I usually tried to keep her out of theatre, she arrived over one morning as I was neutering a particularly large Rottweiler. She chatted away for a few minutes, seemingly oblivious to the whole procedure. Then after a few moments of silence (normally an ominous sign), she blurted out, 'Why are you cutting out the doggy's humps?'

I racked my brains for a suitable answer.

'Well, Roly was being a bit bold,' I finally replied, 'so this just helps him to have better manners.'

At the time, Molly was having an issue with one of the older boys in the local playground, who seemed to delight in terrorising anyone younger or more vulnerable than him. After a few moments of thoughtful silence, during which I thought the matter had been dropped, she continued, 'If you cut Nathan's humps out would that make him have better manners?'

Silently, I thought it sounded like a great idea; I had recently discovered an inner aggression I never knew I possessed, when exposed to any sort of violence – no matter how innocent – towards my children, but reluctantly I told Molly it really only worked for dogs.

With this experience in mind, for the younger-audience school talks, I generally avoided any discussion of humps or any other anatomical details and focused instead on the whole unwanted-puppies issue.

Despite my best intentions, however, I soon discovered that this was totally wasted on the under-tens in general.

'But I would want to *keep* the puppies,' the first child would start.

Carefully, I would begin the explanation of how one puppy would lead to five more, and then five more again.

'But we would keep them *all*,' the next child in line would reassure me.

'And I would love a puppy and I know my friend up the road wants one too,' and within minutes the small handful of children would have successfully rehomed enough puppies to empty the busiest of animal shelters.

The next year, I tried playing a game with them in an attempt to get the message across. I began by picking two children to stand up at the top of the class to be the 'mammy and daddy cat'. Then I would ask three more children to join them, as their kittens. Then each girl kitten would get three new kittens, and this carried on until all the children had been assigned as kittens. The kids were loving it, despite a little bit of inter-sibling squabbling! The next phase of the game didn't go down so well. I asked the first six children to sit down as the ones who had found loving homes with families that would care for them. That was fine. Then the next set of children I sent to one corner representing the ones who would become stray cats. Initially they had great fun hissing and spitting at each other, until I started to describe how some of them would become sick or injured and, with no owner to care for them, some would die. This group didn't look quite so pleased. The next group I then sent to the pound and they were starting to look so tearful that I decided to abandon the whole game before we had to put most of them to sleep and have a total meltdown!

To distract them from their distress, I quickly moved to what I had always found to be the most successful part of the talk. Over the early years, before the onset of digital radiography, I had accumulated several large boxes of radiographs. I also had a special file for the more extraordinary ones. One was of a full-sized red kite that, unusually, had been found dead at sea. As these birds are a protected species, the bird had been brought to me by the wildlife officer for post-mortem examination, which included a radiograph. In the end, the post mortem was not needed, as the radiograph itself was diagnostic. As soon as I raised the still-wet radiograph to the light viewer, the multiple pellets from a shotgun were clearly visible throughout the unfortunate bird's body.

This one was very successful, in particular with the younger kids, as they were so enthralled by the view of the bird, especially when I showed them full-colour pictures of red kites alongside it. Strangely, they seemed not to notice or ever ask about the pellets. With the older classes, however, I would point them out and explain that these birds were a protected species and have a chat about the breeding and reintroduction programme. However one class got ahead of me. As soon as I put up the colour pictures of the bird one of the fifth class boys immediately piped up.

'It's a red kite, Miss. We had two of those flying over the yard and my Dad shot one of them and then we never saw the other one after.'

We never learned, in five years of intensive college lectures, practicals and tutorials how to deal with that one!

Another radiograph that used to go down well, but with slightly less dramatic implications, was one of the knee of a horse. It was of a fifteen-two gelding, on whom I had been asked to carry out a pre-purchase examination. Although the horse was sound on a flexion test, one knee was considerably larger than the other, so I advised a radiograph to rule out any underlying pathology that might potentially cause lameness in time to come. The early history of the horse was unknown, as he had initially come from a dealer's yard. The reason for the thickened joint soon became obvious with the radiograph as the tissue at the front of the knee was full of tiny pieces of stone. The bony structure of the knee is impressive in itself, especially to the uninitiated. This case clearly demonstrated the principle of always taking two radiographs from different angles. In the view taken from the front, or the cranio-caudal view as it is more grandly known, the tiny particles were barely visible as shadows against the bones on the now somewhat fading film. In the lateral view, or the view taken from the side, the stones in front of the bones were obvious. This pair of radiographs always made me feel like a squirming student as I flashed back to images of my college days, standing in front of the great Hester McAllister, our chief radiographer, who simultaneously inspired and terrified generations of veterinary students!

Clearly, the horse had fallen and cut his knee at some stage, but had healed completely, most likely without any sort of veterinary attention and, being a grey horse, the wound had left no visible scarring. In the many years that my client owned the horse after he never showed any ill-effects.

Over the years, I had collected many radiographs of unusual canine fractures. It was always fun to show the picture of the broken bones first – sometimes quite spectacular looking – and then the post-surgical repair, which could look especially dramatic if there were metal bone-plates or pins or wire involved.

I have to admit that I did choose cases that I could follow up with a third radiograph of the fully repaired and functional limb – sometimes with the metal removed, sometimes not, depending on the situation. After seeing how the kids reacted to me making them homeless kittens, I had no intentions of admitting to amputating a leg if the surgical repair failed!

Another radiograph that caused a bit of consternation was one of a mature terrapin, approximately one foot in diameter, who was brought in to me at the Blue Cross clinic in Ballyfermot one night in a large, inauspicious-looking plastic bucket. The unfortunate creature waited patiently in the bucket unknown to us until his turn came. The owners had lost interest as he had grown considerably in size. They had left him out in the garden with only an old dog kennel for shelter against the still-chilly April temperatures. Unsurprisingly, given the time of year, he had stopped eating. They dropped him on the table with the ominous phrase I had come to dread, 'We want you to put him to sleep unless you can find a home for him.'

Although the Blue Cross do not in any way involve themselves in rehoming animals, I decided to bring him home with me. Thankfully, Tommy had a happy ending as the malnutrition and secondary pneumonia that I diagnosed after his radiograph responded well to basic veterinary treatment in the form of antibiotics and rehydration fluids and supplements. Within weeks, he was back in his bucket and on his way to a new home to owners with considerably more reptile experience. His radiograph, however, stayed with us and was always a popular one, as the kids quickly guessed it was a tortoise or indeed a terrapin by of the more avid reptile fanciers. On this occasion, before anyone got a change to guess the correct answer, one guy clearly impressed by the well-rounded body shape yelled out in obvious delight, 'It's Miss Hartigan after eating too many burgers!' The class exploded in eruptions of laughter much to my bewilderment. As there was no teacher present in the room at the time I had to wait until one of the classmates cheerfully informed me that 'Miss Hartigan is the head mistress and she's really fat!'

🐿 🐿 🐿

Probably the most spectacular of my series of school radiographs was of the squirrel that Donal happened to drive past on his way home one bright spring afternoon. Being, in general, a very observant person, he happened to notice what he thought was the dead body of a red squirrel in the ditch. Having a keen interest in nature, he stopped to examine it only to notice that the tiny creature was still warm and breathing, but barely. He gently curled the little body into his woollen hat and brought him straight into the clinic. A rapid clinical examination confirmed that the squirrel was in shock, so I quickly brought him into the theatre and placed him on an oxygen mask. I was able to radiograph the barely conscious form without the sedation that is usually legally required.

His radiographs revealed no abnormalities, or certainly none that were obvious to me with my incredibly limited experience of assessing squirrel radiographs. I began by placing him under a heat lamp, having given him fluid directly into his abdomen, rather than the usual intravenous route. Since he was a wild animal, I was afraid of how he might react if he were to regain consciousness in unfamiliar territory with a fluid line attached to his delicate body. By that evening he had regained consciousness, but clearly had some form of head injury as he was very disorientated.

One fortunate side effect of this head injury was that he became very easy to handle, to the extent that he actually appeared to be tame. In the few days he was with us, he would quite happily climb onto my hand and make his way onto my shoulder, where he would sit contentedly as though I were some unusual species of tree. We filled his hospital unit with various leaves and branches and darkened it with a large towel covering the front, to reduce his stress levels in captivity.

He had started to drink and eat by himself and then on the third morning, when I went in to feed him he was dead. Unfortunately this is an all-too-common outcome with wild animals, even those with apparently minimal injuries. It is often a difficult decision whether to even try treating them, as any human intervention, no matter how sensitively undertaken, is bound to be stressful. A quick and humane euthanasia is often the most realistic option and yet, over the years, a handful of successes have always made me reluctant to do so.

So that's how I acquired the radiograph of a squirrel! And though Barney passed on, he became immortal through his radiograph, which became famous among the primary schools of west Wicklow!

I would usually save it until last, just as the kids were gaining confidence in their skills in identifying animals.

Barney's radiograph was usually greeted with stunned silence. Nine times out of ten the first child brave enough to venture an opinion would cautiously ask, 'Is it a dinosaur?' Nobody would laugh, because everyone was thinking the same thing! Incidentally, that was how Barney acquired his name in his short time with a household of preschool children immersed in Barney the dinosaur!

The most obvious identifying features of a squirrel's skeleton (and possibly also a dinosaur's, I'm not sure!) is the remarkably long canines – very useful for breaking open nuts – and the incredibly long tail, which without being able to the see the bushy fur is very misleading. Nobody ever identified the radiograph as a squirrel, even when I would throw it open to the occasional teacher who would stay for the talk.

In general, those sessions were the more entertaining part of my school talk, which was just as well as it often served me well to get out of a sticky corner. Probably my most traumatic moment of all the school talks was on a day with a very young group of probably five- to eight-year-olds. I had quickly run through the basics of responsible pet ownership, fully aware that realistically, the only bit that grabbed their attention was the fact that round worms looked like spaghetti, while tape worm segments more resemble grains of rice. As I dispensed these nuggets of information, I sent a silent apology to any of the parents who were hoping to serve either carbohydrate for dinner that evening!

After that, things generally deteriorated. I had long since given up on my prepared talk, as I had found that the kids were much more interested in telling about their own pets, their friends' pets, their neighbours' pets, their grannies' pets, even their teddy bear or any other random piece of information that temporarily grabbed their attention.

I prepared myself to stand patiently and be bombarded for the next half hour. One child told me how her granny's dog had run away; another immediately bettered her story with the fact that her granny had died and her dog now lived with them. The next child told me how her cat got 'mashed' – her words, not mine – by a car and broke his leg, and this led to the next child who triumphantly exclaimed that his *brother* had broken his leg. Another little girl bounced up to the front of the class to show me the new bracelet she had been given for her birthday while other random voices filled me in on all the minute details of their busy lives.

I let it all run for a while, until I noticed one small girl over to the side of the room, looking very dejected, I assumed, because she was unable to have her say. At the next millisecond of a gap, I grabbed the moment and, smiling encouragingly at her, asked if she had anything she wanted to tell us. She stared at me silently for a few breaths and then with great big tears rolling down her cheeks told me, 'You killed my dog!'

The silence for which I had previously prayed was now overwhelming. I frantically racked my brains trying to recognise the child, knowing dismally that I had no hope of attaching her to one of many dogs that I had put to sleep over the last few years. Thankfully, having now started, little Jennie recounted to the whole class how Toby had got too old and wasn't able to walk anymore. Through gasps and splutters, she told anyone who cared to listen how her mammy and daddy had rung me to come out to house and when she came back from her friend's house that evening, 'He was dead' she wailed, collapsing into a final sob.

And then I remembered the ancient sheepdog that I had put to sleep a couple of weeks previously. I remembered how peacefully he had drifted off, sleeping in front of the fire, with Brian and Ann, the parents, kneeling on the soft carpet beside him, secure in the knowledge that they were sparing Jenny of the ordeal, by allowing her to stay at a friend's house until the deed was done.

As I knelt on the hard school floor, with my arm around the weeping Jenny, it occurred to me, not for the first time, that final year in veterinary college might be more usefully engaged in studying counselling and psychology than medicine and surgery.

Eventually, the tears ran dry as the rest of the class ran riot until one of the teachers came back and thankfully took control of the rioters. Before I left, Jenny did brighten up significantly as with a tentative smile she told me, 'We're getting another Toby next week,' quickly adding, 'but he won't be the same as the old Toby,' lest I be confused!

That episode did scare me off somewhat from my school talks, so when the National School in Tinahely rang me a few weeks later to enquire whether I would be available, I hesitated.

'We did ring last year, but you were booked up and you said if we rang early this year you would fit us in,' the principal gently reminded me.

Reluctantly I agreed, on condition that a teacher remain in the class with each group.

🐾 🐾 🐾

Hence my sense of trepidation this morning, as I headed down the winding roads to Tinahely, having safely deposited Molly and Fiona at playschool while Jack, now getting hardy as he approached his ninth month, entertained my mother for the morning. Armed with my radiographs and some spot prizes of pens and stickers for responsible pet owners, I arrived in the tiny village, only to realise that though I had passed through on many occasions, I had never actually noticed the National School. After stopping at the local grocery shop for directions, I was soon on my way and within minutes I was pulling into the school grounds.

For all their enthusiasm on the phone, the teachers didn't seem so keen when I arrived. It took me a few minutes to locate a hassled-looking secretary who seemed vaguely put out when I explained that I would take junior infants up to second class in the hall for the first group and then third to sixth class in the second group.

It took a while to assemble the groups and now I was feeling slightly put out as I started thinking of the multitude of other things I could, and probably should, be doing for the next hour and a half. The talks themselves were uneventful, with thankfully no references to obese teachers or discussion of life and death, but by the time I left, having cut the second half short because the hall was needed, I was feeling a bit annoyed. I declined the half-heartedly offered cup of tea.

I was even more annoyed when I got back into the car to find four missed calls and two voicemails, all from the same number.

Quickly I went to my voicemail, wondering what calamity awaited me.

'Hi Gillian, Mary Murphy here, school principal here in Tinahely, just wondering if you are on your way, as the kids are all excitedly waiting for you. Thank you.'

How rude, I thought. I had only been a few minutes late and the principal hadn't even had the manners to greet me, never mind have the kids organised.

The next message.

'Hi there again, Gillian. Sorry to be bothering you. I know you are probably on an emergency call. Just the kids are all assembled here, and some them have even brought their dogs and one little girl has brought her two rabbits and a neighbour's parrot to show you. I think the animals are getting a little stressed, and I was just wondering if I should send them home in case you're not going to make it today. So sorry to bother you,' she ended ever so politely, but sounding a little bit stressed herself.

Through my utter confusion arose the possibility, which sadly turned out to be the reality, that there might in fact be *two* primary schools in the tiny village of Tinahely and that I had barged in to the wrong one demanding to have the classes assembled into the correct groups, never having been invited in the first place.

My first phone call was to Mary Murphy, to apologise profusely to her for the confusion and to suggest that, yes, the animals would be best returned to their rightful homes for another day, as I now had just less than half an hour to get to the playschool for my children.

Then humbly I rang the second school, to again apologise profusely for the confusion, and thank them most graciously for their welcome and for accommodating my unexpected arrival.

It was at that stage I decided that, with three children of my own to look after, my time for school talks was over!

CHAPTER 6

THE MISSION EXPANDS

Although the eight-foot-by-eight-foot utility room and the adjacent portacabin had been more than sufficient, though somewhat intrusive on family life, for the opening years of Clover Hill Veterinary Clinic, it was not long before it became apparent that we needed to expand. I had genuinely planned on setting up from home only until Jack was ready for school, and then, in my words, I was going to get a 'real job' in a mixed-animal practice. But of course life never reads the manual we write for ourselves, so, not long after Jack's first birthday, it became apparent that I now had a 'real job' in a rapidly expanding dedicated small animal practice.

The 'waiting room' for the clinic, consisted of clients queuing around the gravel driveway of the house and there were increasingly frequent evenings when it looked like we would have to add a second lane! Equally, the consulting room that doubled as a theatre, apart from the time spent in meticulously cleaning the room between each job change, was just becoming inadequate.

In fairness to the clients, I genuinely don't ever remember anyone complaining about the inconvenience. From day one, I was simply overwhelmed by the sheer enthusiasm of the clients and put all my effort into providing the best possible care for their furry family members and their owners too, determined not to compromise patient care in our tiny facilities. And it had paid off. Clients came and then their relations came and then their friends came and still they kept coming. At the time we opened, it was deemed unprofessional for veterinary professionals to advertise and without this, one of the local planners had advised that setting up in such a remote area – up a windy road through the woods, where the access consisted of a narrow track with grass growing up the middle – would be madness. But then she too became a client, as did her extended family and friends, and she was delighted to be proved wrong.

In the winter months, the clinic had to run around the weather forecast and special midday clinics – just at the time when I was due to collect the kids from school – had to be added for elderly people who didn't fancy driving up the twisty roadway on a dark evening. As the months went by, we continually adjusted and adapted to the needs of a practice that was growing at a somewhat alarming rate.

So, far from getting myself ready to join one of the local practices, I was back with a pen and paper, sketching, converting our existing farm shed, which comfortably housed a handful of retired equine pensioners, along with the infamous

Robo, the kids' pony. We started by looking at converting half the shed and moving the horses to the other half, but then, as my plans became more adventurous, the half for the veterinary practice extended into the far side, and the horses got sketched into an adjoining building. We were due to meet with Donal Kavanagh, who had built the original shed, to see about building a new shed for the horses before we started evicting them. The afternoon of the meeting, we were out the front with the kids when one of the neighbour farmers drove up the windy road. As usual on seeing us outside, the big red truck pulled to a halt and Molly, still enthusiastic about inviting the entire neighbourhood in for a cup of tea, ran in to boil the kettle. It was a familiar scene as we had come to know John Armstong well in the years since we had moved to the rural village of Glenealy.

I had first met John high up on hill farm, somewhere between Laragh and Glendalough, back in my pre-children days when I was working in Riverside Veterinary Clinic. The same red truck was parked outside the shale driveway of an old farmyard, and I followed him up the rough laneway that looked like it was just going to disappear into the misty mountaintop. It was only when we reached the semi-derelict shed and I saw the two bachelor farmers who actually owned the property that I realised that John had just come along to help. It didn't take long to realise why I might need help as I peered into the dark shed to see three loose bullocks charging around in utter confusion at being penned into the tiny building with no natural daylight. Over the indignant bawling of the cattle, I nervously asked where the crush was, as I had come to TB test the three bullocks – the entire stock of the elderly brothers.

John chuckled gently at my naive question and, without answering, started sliding the rusty bolt and heaving open the door that was wedged in what looked like generations of old manure. Temporarily stunned by the stream of daylight that shone uninvited to the dark corners of the shed, the cattle stood snorting at us as I looked on in bewilderment, wondering how I was supposed to clip and inject these animals, never mind read their muck-caked tags. Still John said nothing. As my eyes gradually accustomed to the dim light, I noticed a rusty farm gate in the corner, tied with an old rope to what once was the outline of a window frame. As he moved quietly between the cattle, he pulled the gate, or what was left of it, around, producing what, I assumed, was to be the crush. It didn't escape my notice that neither Mick nor Jimmy, the bachelor brothers, chose to join us as I hesitantly made my way to the far corner, hoping to persuade the steaming beasts into the makeshift crush.

As there wasn't much space, the first two actually ran into it without noticing, and I tried to steady my hand as I gave a cursory clip to the neck in two areas before injecting the sites. By the time I got to the second bullock, the first was three-quarters of the way out the front. He made a lunge over the gate, landing halfway over it and balancing precariously, before the whole thing collapsed, the dusty rope easily surrendering to the weight. I desperately jabbed the needle into my second patient, just as he too joined in the great escape, scrambling awkwardly over what remained of the gate.

Without any visible signs of dismay, John quietly set about setting up the gate once more and, unknotting the remains of the freighting rope, managed to somewhat secure the temporary crush. Having seen the frolics of the first two, the last remaining bullock was having none of it. He wheeled from side to side, carefully keeping himself behind his braver brother every time we approached. The heavy breath of cattle was soon matched by my own as we repeatedly tried to anticipate the movement of the reluctant beast as he repeatedly dashed out from the gate just when we thought we had him, lashing out on the last occasion and taking a bar of the rusty gate with him as he galloped by. However, far from getting irate with the bullock and resorting to shouting and roaring to further wind him up, as many farmers I had worked with would have done, John stayed calm and patiently watched and waited until, finally, the reluctant bullock almost accidently ended up between the crush and the wall. In a flash, I reached over the remaining bars and clipped and injected before the bullock had worked out his escape route.

It was only as we were reversing out the door, keeping a

watch on the three eyeballing us from the far corner, that it occurred to me that I hadn't recorded the tag numbers. Not only that, but my little blue book in which all the data was to be written was lying open, face-down on the well-rotted floor. Cautiously easing my way forward, I used an old pitchfork to pull it towards me, not wanting to further offend the bullocks by invading their territory once more. The pencil had long since disappeared, unlikely ever to see the light of day again. By the state of the tags on the cattle's ears, it was unlikely that I would have been able to read them anyway, so I had to reply on Mick's reassurance as he read out their supposed numbers from an old piece of paper which he pulled out of his back pocket.

John laughed easily as we made our way back down the narrow laneway. 'Well, thank God they weren't heifers or we would have had some fun getting blood sample,' I said, catching my breath to keep up with him.

'Ah, sure we would have managed that too,' he replied. Little did I know at the time that over the following months I would meet John again and again in many such situations. Anywhere there was a batchelor or a spinster farmer, or an elderly uncle, or a yard that was somewhat less than adequate, John would quietly appear, whether for a planned TB test or a late-night calving, he seemed to have an uncanny ability to turn up just when he was needed. Although I was always delighted to see the familiar red truck, it usually meant there was some sort of hardship in store!

Despite the fact that he had his own considerable dairy herd and sheep flock, for the first six months in Riverside, I never once saw a call out to John's yard in the day-book. Obviously all the experience in handling everyone else's veterinary issues had left him well equipped to handle his own. With that in mind, I was a little anxious when Seamus rang me one afternoon to say there was a call to go to a calving for John Armstrong. I first assumed it was in some derelict hill farm, and initially felt slightly more enthusiastic when Seamus told me it was in John's own yard – but only for a few moments, until it dawned on me that if John needed help calving a cow, it was not going to be straightforward.

As though reading my thoughts, Seamus confirmed my anxiety as he added, 'I can't ever remember getting a call to a calving to Armstrong's before. I'm tied up testing here for the next hour or so. Go out and give it a go and when you get stuck, ring me. I'll get finished up here and go out and give you a hand.'

Despite his well-intentioned offer, the automatic assumption that I wouldn't be able to do it only made me more determined to succeed, totally dissolving any previous fears I might have had.

As I drove down the long, well-maintained driveway, I was thrilled to see, far from the dilapidated sheds where I usually encountered him, a modern milking parlour, a spacious well-bedded shed and a well-planned cattle crush.

And again, contrary to our usual encounters, everything was ready and waiting, without the usual delay of having to find the farmer, or go and herd up the cattle, or wait for the water to boil on the old stove.

If John looked disappointed to see me instead of Seamus, he didn't show it; I silently hoped I wouldn't let him down. The well-conditioned Friesian cow stood patiently as I inserted my lubricated, gloved hand to feel two tiny hooves in the birth canal. Initially everything seemed okay, and I was pleasantly surprised to find that everything felt fresh and not, as is often the case, like someone had been trying for the last hour without any success.

'I put my hand in, but when I felt things weren't right, I just called Seamus straight away without messing around any further,' John told me, as though reading my mind.

And of course, he was right. Although the front feet were well positioned, when I felt back for the nose to follow on, it was not there. As the cow was quite roomy, I was able to get back past the legs and reach down into the uterus, where I could feel the head of the calf, arching away from me. As the calf was relatively small, I thought it would be easy enough to pull the head around into the birth canal, and then deliver it in its rightful position along with the tiny hooves. But after a few unsuccessful attempts, I realised that it was not going to be so simple. Far from being able to pull the head around, the neck was stiff and hard and I knew that not only was the calf dead, but it also had some sort of deformity that was preventing a normal delivery. It's always more difficult to deliver a dead animal that a live one, but in this case I knew it was going to be trickier than usual, as the deformity might indicate the need for a Caesarean section – always a last resort with a dead calf.

Seamus's offer of help echoed in my mind, but then (I hope out of concern for the cow and not out of my own stubbornness) I decided I might as well give it a go. Working in reverse order from a normal calving, I tried to push the hooves and front legs back out of the birth canal, hoping to make room to bring the head through on its own. Although this would never usually work – and many a difficult calving is simply because the head has come through without the legs – in this case, I felt that the tiny frame of the lifeless animal just might make it through with the legs back, not having any sizeable shoulders to block the birth canal.

After a few failed attempts to then pull the head forward, I hooked a calving rope around the lower jaw, not having to concern myself about the risk of fracturing the delicate bones. Using as much force as I was comfortable with, I painstakingly worked the deformed head into the birth canal. By rotating the body from side to side to get the shoulders through, the calf was eventually slithered through with the last pull.

We were silent as we watched the lifeless form lying on the straw. It was clear that it was grossly deformed and would never have been compatible with life. The cow nuzzled it silently, clearly aware that the calf was dead. It was a sad scene, but at least we had avoided the Caesarean section.

By the time Seamus rang to say he was on his way over, we were sitting down in the homely kitchen, having the first of very many cups of tea that I would have there over the following years. As I bit into one of Margaret's fresh buns, I relayed to Seamus the details of the delivery, and he seemed somewhat taken aback that his assistance had not been required.

It was a few years after that episode that Donal and I were looking at houses to buy in the Wicklow area, needing to upsize our current location due to the then imminent arrival of Molly. When we went to look at the house that we later went on to live in, I pointed John's yard out to Donal as we drove by. He had heard many stories of the our hillside encounters and felt as though he knew him as well as I did. I noted with interest that day that the entrance to John's yard was exactly one mile from our own new entrance.

Before we moved, I had rung John to ask him who I could get to fence the property and a few other such jobs. On the day we arrived with our collection of ponies, the Jersey cow, the three dogs and, of course, three-month-old Molly, he arrived in with a batch of fresh buns from Margaret. And after that it sort of evolved as he would often pass by during the day and drop in for chat so that by the time Fiona and then Jack arrived on the scene they never knew anything other than him being a part of the family.

The long-standing joke about 'John's chair' in the kitchen went back to before Fiona had started playschool – we went to our local furniture shop to buy a new table and chairs for the kitchen, as it seemed to be the central point in our house. When the assistant asked how many people were in the house, Fiona instantly demanded six chairs – one for each of us, including John.

When we went on our first holiday, it was John who minded the collection of ponies, the cow, the dogs and cats, the fish and even the tortoise. A far cry from the steaming bullocks up in Laragh!

John was well involved in the setting up of the practice, and although he had his doubts about a small-animal practice ever succeeding in a rural area, he was always ready to help in any way.

So, on the afternoon that Donal Kavanagh was coming up to discuss building another shed so that we could move the practice, we asked John to drop in too, if he was passing, as having worked with his father as a builder before his farming days, he had a good insight into what would need to be done and would also have many contacts of reputable builders in the area.

With the kids more or less settled in bed, we sat around the kitchen table – myself, Donal, John and Donal Kavanagh – and roughly drafted a plan to add on to the existing shed, leaving the original thirty-by-thirty-foot building to become the new veterinary surgery (giving us back our utility room, taking the washing machine and dryer for all the household washing and the surgery from the bathroom back to the utility room, and hopefully giving us a little more space while allowing the practice the room it needed to expand).

Donal Kavanagh headed off to work on a price for his end of things, while myself, Donal and John sat late into the night looking at what would be needed to do the internal conversions.

Although we already knew a great builder who had done work for us in our previous home, he now lived quite a distance away and we reckoned his price would be beyond what we could realistically afford. John thought about it for a bit and threw around a few names, but didn't seem entirely happy with any of them. He was clearly deep in thought and didn't seem in a hurry to go home. Just as he was heading out the door, he casually mentioned that he might, once Donal had the floor in the original shed, start laying a few blocks until he came up with someone, if that would be okay with us. We were slightly stunned – although he had taken early retirement he was probably busier than ever, as always helping out and appearing in all variety of places that you wouldn't expect to meet him. Nonetheless we were delighted that everything seemed to be taking shape and Clover Hill Veterinary Clinic was going to get a new home.

CHAPTER 7

DAFFODIL LADY

At first, Jenny seemed like just one of those clients who I would meet occasionally as they passed through my life without ever making much of an impact. With some clients, you recognise their arrival by the sound of their dogs yapping. Jenny, I always recognised by the sound of her much-abused car – an ancient Toyota Corolla in faded rusty red that always seemed to have more health issues than her dog.

Jenny, like myself, had little respect for her vehicle, dragging its aged body down the motorway from Dublin despite an overheating engine, to check a minor irritation in her little shih-tzu's ear. I wasn't in a position to criticize, as every time I called into our local garage to give Jessie her monthly joint injection, Pat Driver, the mechanic, would look up at me from under his glasses and quietly ask, 'Have you checked the car for oil lately?' The question was futile, as the current pace of my life did not allow for such indulgences to myself, never mind the car. So, over time, we came to an unwritten agreement that I would keep Jessie, his beloved dog, up to date with her vaccinations and worm doses, while Pat would look after the car. Jessie never did seem terribly enthusiastic about the arrangement; I usually just about caught sight of the tail end of her slinking off as I pulled into the yard but, despite her reluctance, both she and the car kept going very well for a long time.

🦎 🦎 🦎

As always, Jenny's consultation was preceded by a trip to the hose attached to the wall outside the clinic. The engine steamed and hissed as she opened the bonnet of the car to refill the water container. The reason she travelled such a distance to me was that at the time, we were a referral practice for the Blue Cross, though it was questionable whether it was actually cheaper to pay the price of the petrol and the damages to the car than to go to her local practice.

Bella was an itchy type and, over the time I knew her, always suffered some degree of skin allergy and an ongoing ear irritation. Due to Jenny's meagre finances, we were always only just about able to keep it under some sort of control, without ever being able to get to the root of the problem. Expensive medications and diets were way beyond her budget, but she had a big heart and would meticulously cook individual meals for Bella, probably of better quality than the food she ate herself. In her own words, Jenny always had 'plenty of time' on her hands – a concept that seemed so totally alien to me at the time – and so Bella's coat was always well-groomed and in as good a condition as could be expected with her allergies.

The ongoing nature of Bella's condition meant that I saw Jenny quite regularly. Maybe it was the regularity of her visits that strained her poor car to its utter limits, so increasingly Jenny might arrive an hour or two after her appointed time, usually on an evening where Donal was out so I would be on my own at home with the kids by the time she announced her arrival accompanied by loud protests from her heroic car. Her consultations were usually interrupted by my having to take something off the cooker, or rescue Fiona and Jack from some over enthusiastic encounter.

Far from being apologetic about her untimely arrival, Jenny seemed put out by my not-quite-undivided attention, and rolled her eyes every time the door opened from the house or the noise from the kitchen raised by a few decibels. I used to console myself that the time I spent working and away from doing all the things I felt I should have been doing with the kids would in time be justified by earning enough to provide a reasonable standard of living and potentially paying their college fees. Unfortunately, in Jenny's case, I couldn't use this argument as not only did she regularly leave me short of the already-subsidised fee, but I also sometimes had to give her 'a loan' to pay for her petrol to get home.

On one occasion, Bella's ears had flared beyond the levels of ear drops and tablets, so I admitted her for sedation and a more thorough investigation. Jenny was not put out in any way by the fact that I would need to keep Bella for a few hours until the sedation wore off. I suggested a local coffee shop, but with the somewhat limited mileage left in the car, Jenny opted to sit in the car.

It felt rude to leave her sitting there, but she assured me she had an old newspaper and could occupy herself. I didn't bother discussing the extra cost over the usual visit fee; Bella was in so much discomfort that I just couldn't send her home without doing something to alleviate her condition. I sedated the little dog immediately, as she seemed quite anxious at the separation from her full-time companion. Jenny took Bella everywhere.

'If she's not invited, then I simply won't go,' she told me, clearly in a position to commit to her life as an eccentric spinster. I saw a few more clients before Bella was sleepy enough for me to examine the ear properly. I was with great relief that I gently plucked big clumps of matted hair from the delicate ear canal. Although I knew from the scarring in the narrowed ear canal that the relief would only be temporary, at least Bella would wake up feeling better.

To save Jenny any extra delay, instead of letting Bella sleep off the sedation I decided to give her an antidote so that she would wake up within a few minutes. When I went to fill Jenny in on her progress, she had disappeared. As it was a beautiful morning, I decided she had gone off for a walk, but when she hadn't come back over two hours later, I was beginning to worry.

As it was approaching playschool pick up time I had no option but to lock up and head out the road to collect Fiona and Jack, and get them home for a quick snack, before collecting Molly from the dizzying heights of senior infants in the local national school at two. The middle of the day was always a tight period, with even minutes of a delay throwing the finely tuned system out of control. As though innately sensing my sense of urgency, Fiona and Jack chose to go in extra slow motion. The beans were too hot. The butter wasn't spread properly on the toast and a list of other crises to the mind of a toddler. A full glass of milk spewed out across the kitchen floor just as Jenny returned. For once she was unannounced as on foot, and, seeing the locked back door to the surgery, she poked her head in the kitchen window.

Jack screamed in fright at the head in the window while Fiona took the opportunity to dance up and down, shrieking with delight as the milk splashed beneath her pink boots.

I had to leave Jenny as I piled the reluctant pair back into the car to race down to the, thankfully, very local primary school. Molly was full of news about a new girl in the class, but I only half heard her, as I planned to dish out a packet of rice cakes in front of a video while I discharged Bella, wondering why Jenny could never actually come at a time I was organised.

Having gone through Bella's discharge medications with Jenny, I went to hand her the bill. Jenny apologised and ran back out to the car. She arrived back with a large bunch of daffodils, which had clearly been roughly pulled from their roots and tied in what looked like an old tissue.

'I knew there would be an extra charge, but I had nothing on me so I got you these,' she said, offering me the raggy bunch of half-bloomed flowers. I accepted them graciously, trying not to wonder whether Coillte or one of the neighbours' gardens had donated them.

Just as we loaded Bella into the car, a shrick erupted from the sitting room, breaking the short peaceful silence.

'You know,' Jenny said to me, cranking down the car window as the engine reluctantly spluttered to some sort of life. 'You might think you're some sort of super woman, but you're not. You might think you can do it all, but you're neglecting those children.' With that she reversed out of the drive way, and turned up the windy road, leaving a thick trail of smoke behind her.

I was momentarily stunned, but only for an instant, as I then had to pull myself together to pick up the pieces of the latest calamity in the sitting room.

It was evening before I actually had time to allow her words to register. I couldn't help but feel that maybe she was right. When I had first set up the practice, it was purely because I could not get a job in mixed practice with a young baby. Night work and out-of-hours calls in a large-animal practice and all it entailed meant that I had decided to work from home, purely so that I would be there while the kids were small. I had always planned on returning to mixed practice once Jack was old enough to go to school.

Some of the clients also noticed how increasingly busy I was becoming. One elderly lady came to visit with her two geriatric dogs, purely to register them with the practice as a friend had recommended us. She was an absolute lady and we chatted for some time about her two 'boys' and some people we knew in common. When I met the friend who had first recommended us she told me that Meryl had loved the practice, but decided not to register with as I, in her words, 'looked utterly exhausted'.

Although slightly taken aback, I was touched by her concern. Although I had never until that day, to my knowledge, laid eyes on Meryl, it seemed in the weeks that followed, that we were destined to 'stalk' each other, as we began to bump into each other in all sorts of unusual places: in a petrol station, at the post office, passing by the local bookshop. We followed each other all around Wicklow over a period of about two weeks. That Friday evening, we met at the check-out in Lidl. As I unpacked my piled-high groceries, I noticed a young mother with two small children behind me with only a handful of items. As I was unusually child-free that evening, I told her to go ahead of me. As she thanked me and passed me by, the man behind her snorted indignantly.

'Just because you have all the time in the world to do your shopping, it doesn't mean the rest of us have all day to spend in here.'

I hadn't noticed Meryl standing at the till beside me, but she had overheard the comment and was having none of it.

'Young man,' she said, although he was clearly in his sixties, 'this lady is probably the busiest person you or I will ever meet.' There was a silence from the usually bleary-eyed shoppers, as Meryl had spoken in tones loud enough for everyone to hear.

The man looked away. Picking up his basket, he shuffled off to a till at the far end of the shop, which incidentally had a much longer queue.

Meryl did end up becoming not only a client, but also a friend as, over the years, I tended to her elderly pensioners. We sat in her elegant back kitchen when, several months apart, I was called to assist with the passing of first one, then the other of her beloved pensioners, freeing them from the suffering of bladder cancer in the case of one, and simple old age in the other. Although devastated, Meryl was grateful that her boys' endings had been so peaceful.

'I hope when my time comes,' she whispered to me, her then-frail hand holding mine, 'that you will be there too.'

Some years later, I discovered by means of a phone call from a kindly neighbour that Meryl was in her final days. Politely ignoring the 'no visitors' sign, remembering her request that day in her kitchen, I went up one evening to sit with Meryl, sadly not in her comfortable kitchen, but lying in a hospital bed, and thought back to the feisty lady that was too concerned to come to me as I looked too tired.

She was not conscious as I sat and chatted to her, but deep down, I felt her presence was still there and that she knew I was there too. After a while, Brian O'Reilly, her local rector, arrived also and we sat for some time either side of her, reminiscing about old stories from the time we had known her. At one stage, one of her machines started to beep and, resisting the urge to get up and check it, we waited patiently for the nurse on duty to come in. Having reset the machine, she turned to myself and the Rev. Brian and kindly asked if we were relations. Brian immediately stood up and introduced himself as the Rector. She shook his hand warmly and asked was I a relation. 'Oh, no,' I replied without thinking. 'I'm Meryl's vet.' Despite the nurse's confusion, we all roared laughing and I feel sure that Mcryl was highly amused to be laid out, flanked by the Rector and the vet in her dying days.

In her time, and although Meryl had no children herself, she had always reassured me that our children were so lucky to be brought up in veterinary practice. She seemed to see the positives and the ways in which it enriched their slightly chaotic lives. She was always amused to see them flitting through the practice with an assortment of animals, and watched with great interest as they grew and developed their own interests over the years.

I suppose it's something that every working mother wrestles with, and there were days and moments where I felt I had got it badly wrong. Ken, the courier, brought it home clearly to me on one occasion in particular; I had been up sporadically through every night of the preceding week, as the kids and the clients seemed to have a hidden rota, carefully taking it in turns to ensure that I never got a night of uninterrupted sleep. Ken was unfortunate enough to have to make his way up the windy bends through the woods to the practice most days of the week, delivering orders, and became well known to the kids. Molly would, in anticipation of his daily drop offs, be waiting at the gate to offer him the customary 'cup of tea', which he always politely declined.

He usually dropped the parcels in the back door, but on this day, I was unusually late opening up. I had dragged myself out of bed well after when I should have got up, and barked grumpily at the kids when they started wrestling with each other over some unknown offense. It was one of those days when I just knew I would have to hold it together for a few hours until the morning blues passed and my inner night owl kicked in. I couldn't find the keys when Ken rang at the back door. When I finally managed to open the door, and peered out at him through bleary eyes, I was surprised to see him standing on the doorstep, tears streaming down his face.

'I'm sorry,' he said. Taking a deep breath between peals of laughter. 'I went to the front door, but the little one opened it and said you were in a bad mood, so I wasn't to talk to you or I would make you cry!'

And cry he did – laughing so hard! Thankfully he himself had four children much the same age as ours, so he didn't ring Childline on the way out, but hopefully rang his wife to make her feel better.

Despite my self-questioning, there were many good times too. Our house was always a noisy house, filled with people and dogs and cats, and even the goats sometimes chose to break in. The old Shetland pony made it as far as the sitting room one afternoon. As a child, with my allergies, despite my protest, pets were limited. In our house, we made up for it and probably even went overboard. Every bed had a dog as well as a child. The house was never tidy, but well-messed from being lived in!

The hens and ducks were tamed thanks mainly to Fiona's intervention, although the geese never really joined in. Clients became used to being met by a trio of geese in the driveway; we eventually had to rehome them to a client with a large lake after the gander got a little over excited in the middle of an evening clinic during breeding season. In the early days, before increasing client numbers made it cost-prohibitive, we used to make Christmas cards with pictures of our pets. When the geese featured one year, the local printers rang just to double check whether the cards were for the butchers or the vets?

One afternoon in particular, I thought that maybe living in a veterinary practice was not such a bad upbringing for a child.

I could hear the three kids in high glee as we finished up the clinic one afternoon. I knew Donal was home, so I didn't have to check up on them, but I did wonder what they were up to that was causing such mirth and merriment.

When I did get out to see them, it took a few minutes to work out what was going on. Molly's rocking horse lay stretched on his side on the grassy area in front of the clinic, just at the point where the clients drive in and out. Robo the rocking horse was named after her first pony, the only word she would say in public for about the first eighteen months of her life, much to the concern of the local health nurse and GP.

Apparently, Robo (the rocking horse) had been jumping a big jump, but got run over by a randomly passing unicorn. I listened carefully as they explained this to me, all of them talking at once. Anyway, the unicorn had apparently inflicted a severe wound, and now the luckless Robo required surgery. Unsure how to anaesthetise him, but having seen me placing the gas mask over our furry patient's heads, the three had come up with a plan and, quickly acquiring one of Donal's thick walking socks, assured each other that the smell would be enough to anesthetise the horse! So the horse lay on his side, enormous sock hanging over his muzzle, while Molly, as chief surgeon, wrapped the front limb in layers of vetwrap – not to be found in any children's toy shop – while Fiona monitored the horse with the stethoscope and Jack sat on the horse's head just in case.

The three aspiring surgeons drew much entertainment out ofthe entire procedure, while later that evening I went to return the recovered horse to his bedroom, the used vetwrap to the clinical waste bin and the anaesthetic mask to the dirty clothes basket!

🪶 🪶 🪶

But it wasn't only their toys that stirred their imaginations. Despite the craziness of life in a veterinary practice, the live animals always provided much scope for real entertainment and life learning.

Late one night, long past the time when the three were soundly asleep, I went to top up the horses' feed and check the small terrier in the clinic recovering from a nasty bite wound.

As I pulled over the door of the hay shed, I heard a tiny sound over the loud hissing of the goose, who had patiently sat on clutches of eggs over three breeding seasons, but never actually managed to hatch any. I listened again and knew instantly that at last, the goose's patience was being rewarded. Carefully holding her beneath her head, I looked under to see a tiny, wet body still sitting in the half-opened egg. Goose eggs do not hatch as easily as hen or duck eggs and they often need assistance to break out of the thick shell.

Although it was late and probably against the guidance of any parenting or child-sleep manual, I raced over to the house and, wrapping the kids up in warm fleecy jumpers and boots, brought them over, sleepy-eyed, to the shed. They were unusually hushed as I sat them up on the hay bale and gently withdrew the half-hatched gosling from its shell. Their eyes lit up in total awe as the little wet body began to shake itself and chirped loudly, demanding that I replace him with his anxious mother. We spent almost an hour there as three more of the large eggs began to hatch, and with each one they watched as the little body emerged from its cocoon to start a new life.

Although, many times over the years, I have thought about the daffodil lady and oftentimes agreed with her, on that magical star-filled night, I felt that maybe I wasn't doing such a bad job.

CHAPTER 8

AN UNEXPECTED SITE INSPECTION

Before starting to build the new premises, life seemed full-on – running a twenty-four/seven on-call practice out of a utility room with three pre-school children. So taking the practice out of the house seemed like a good idea; at least my nightly routine would no longer include dividing the soiled vet beds from the kids' clothes to wash separately in the washing machine that resided in the bathroom (with the tumble dryer perched precariously on top as the utility room was otherwise occupied). I used to put on a load going to bed and hope it would be finished before Jack woke in the night so I could get another load on once he had settled. Most people store shoes or spare blankets under their beds. Ours was packed with sacks of dog food as our tiny premises didn't stretch to holding more than two or three sacks at a go.

Competition was fierce in the world of dog food sales, and when one of the sales reps saw our potential for growth, he offered me a weekend away if I would commit to their food for the next twelve months; I asked him if he would babysit the kids some Friday night instead, but he declined. Sales reps are inevitably a part of any business. In the early days, some of them went out of their way to help me, going beyond the call of duty to get me up and running, clearly in awe or perhaps in shock, watching me try to balance the practice with the toddlers. Some, however, clearly didn't see past their own sales figures, and would call in unannounced when I was trying to stitch up the morning's bitch spay before hurrying to collect the kids from playschool.

So the idea of having a separate premises from which to run the practice was not only appealing, but rapidly becoming essential. With John lined up to supervise the entire project, things began to happen.

Once Donal Kavanagh and his sons had finished building on the new section to rehome our collection of horses, goats and poultry, we started working on dismantling the interiors of the old shed that was to be transformed into the practice. From then on, the day's veterinary work ended to be followed by moving across the fence to the yard to see what progress had been made over the day and to plan for the next step.

I was lucky that in my early days of working I had been involved in numerous animal welfare groups, and been involved in the design of building new premises. Also from my locum days, I had developed ideas of what worked and what didn't. Long winter evenings had been spent sketching and re-sketching my ideal premises into the outline of the old stables. Compromises had to be made, but in the end I was satisfied. The consulting room was spacious, but not too big. The waiting room was to be open and large enough to separate predator from prey! Even more importantly, the cattery and kennels were in separate, soundproof rooms, ensuring that the in-patients would not be sharing airspace with some terrifying inmate.

The theatre was a separate room and had direct access to the radiography room – useful during orthopaedic surgery. I was also happy to have a large treatment room, where animals would be prepared for theatre and other work-ups and diagnostic tests could be carried out. The ultrasound and blood machines, I knew, were excessive at the moment for the size of the practice, but equally I knew they were essential for the quality of care I wanted to offer our patients. I could only hope that by putting everything in place, patients would come. As the sketches were drawn and redrawn, the kids were happy to fill them with their own drawings of ponies and kittens and unicorns and penguins and snow leopards. It was looking like Clover Hill Veterinary Clinic would be an exciting place to work!

Once the physical work began, things got even more hectic. Donal would leave for work before six, leaving me to organise the kids for the morning. Once the girls were in playschool, and Jack with a child minder, I would try to fit a day's work into the morning. Over the day, we would keep in touch to see which of us could collect the kids at lunchtime and which would keep working.

From there, the afternoon would be spent between the kids and the surgery, while Donal doubled as a labourer, or bricklayer, or delivery man, or any of the endless roles that were needed to keep up with John as he meticulously made his way through the building of the surgery. The clients were all interested in the building, work which was clearly visible from the current surgery. Occasionally, I would bring them over and give them a preliminary tour; the clients, as much as us, were eagerly anticipating the big move. The tiny eight-foot -by-eight-foot consulting room from which the entire practice was operating at the time was feeling smaller and smaller as the practice got busier and busier.

It was exciting to watch the building grow. When the walls had been laid to a height of three bricks all around, I took to walking around it, imagining myself bringing a dog through this doorway on a trolley, or an owner through another doorway. I could see in my mind how it would all look once complete. The kids, of course, saw it as a massive playground, and Jack, not yet two years old, became a member of the building crew when Donal Kavanagh arrived one day with a delivery of blocks and a kid's dumper truck for Jack.

Technically, Jack was the first person to work on developing the new premises. Although only eighteen months by the time we got to this stage of the building work, he had developed an interest in anything involving mass destruction. When the old internal walls that had divided the ponies had to be knocked down, Jack was the first in with the hammer (under Donal and John's watchful supervision) to begin the demolition act! The already-crumbling block bricks easily succumbed to the hammer, which he swung with an enthusiasm that made me have serious concerns about his teenage years!

It was hard to catch your breath at times, there was so much going on. One evening, when, thankfully, the kids were chilling in front of a DVD, I was just seeing the last few appointments for the evening clinic while John and Donal were preparing for the next day's jobs. In the distance, I thought I heard some cattle roaring, but being surrounded by field of sucklers this was not an unusual sound on the breezy spring evening.

While I injected the elderly Labrador, whose hips were slowing him down more than his head, I was sure the sound was getting louder. Even Rollo's ears pricked up as I helped heave his overweight body into the back of the car. My last patient for the evening was Nina, a dainty poodle. Her owner was waiting nervously in the car, terrified of meeting any other dogs with her beloved Nina (who I actually suspected would be quite happy to take on her fellow canines). I beckoned them in and the car door had only shut when I suddenly realised that the roar of cattle was even closer than I had thought; within seconds I could hear the unmistakable sound of hooves on the gravel driveway coming around the back of the surgery.

An elderly and much respected professor of ours from college days used to say 'when you hear the sounds of hooves, think horses not zebrae', meaning common things are common. I couldn't help thinking of him in those split seconds. As the first head appeared at speed, heading directly for Nina in her trembling owner's arms, I didn't waste any more time but threw my arms around the two of them and shoved them in the surgery door just as the cattle were upon us. As I slammed the door shut behind my client, I swung around to try to stop the unlikely visitors, but clearly the sight of me manhandling a body through the surgery door had spooked them and they spun around, showers of gravel flying in all directions, and ran back straight towards the fence separating the house from what was to become the new surgery. They hesitated for a split second looking as though they were going to jump, but then, in a frenzy of excitement, just ran straight through the flimsy fence designed for dogs and toddlers not five-hundred kilo cattle.

John and Donal had heard the noise and came out to see what was going on. On seeing the men in their path, the three adventurous bullocks spun past them and in through the door of the surgery. The neat rows of blocks, three bricks high, laying out the outline of the rooms in the new surgery served as perfect hurdling grounds as they galloped from room to room, luckily clearing each tiny wall instead of taking it with them. In their excitement, streams of hot steamy faeces sprayed out of them, as they completed another lap of the building before charging back out into the front field.

Luckily by then, Donal had had time to shut the main gates and between us we were able to curtail them in the front field while John made a few phone calls. We discovered that Sean Cooney, a local farmer, had just returned from the mart with his new charges who, instead of running down the ramp into the well-prepared shed, had managed to go through the side barriers and were last seen heading at speed down the laneway. As he lived around the corner, it was only a matter of minutes before we heard the rattle of the cattle trailer and between us, and ably assisted by his daughter Izzy Cooney, we herded the escapees back into the trailer. It was only then, with the cattle safely loaded, that I remembered Nina and her owner, stuffed into the tiny consulting room at the house. I hopped what remained of the fence dividing the house from the new surgery and found Linda waiting, surprisingly calmly, in the consulting room, Nina still clutched in her arms.

'I didn't know you treated large animals as well,' was her only comment. She clearly thought that the three bullocks had simply been waiting their turn.

It wasn't the only time we had uninvited patients at the clinic – on several occasions over the years random animals arrived in to the clinic. My favourite of all guests arrived late one night as I was going to check on a dog who had cut himself badly while out chasing a stick in the woods. He had severed a vessel and was bleeding profusely, so despite the hour I took him into theatre and cauterised the wounds under anaesthetic. I came back to check on him well after midnight. As I went to unlock the back door, I had a feeling of being watched and as I looked into the darkness, there stood a deer, not six feet from me in the trees at the back of the surgery. We stood staring at each other for some time before I gently asked her, 'Do you have an appointment?' She blinked and then turned and ran, clearly unwilling to surrender herself to my skills.

Patient care was, of course, the priority for every decision in the design and building of the surgery. When the walls of the theatre were being built, a five-centimetre hole had to be drilled in the wall near the ground, to allow the outlet of the anaesthetic machine to be passed through. John was concerned that the hole would allow rats in, and so fitted a vent on the outside of the wall. But I was more concerned about rats or mice or chipmunks or other tiny patients getting out! The plans had to be revised yet again!

For the year or more that it took to build the surgery, free time or any sort of a social life were something that happened to other people. We hadn't taken a holiday in years, and it didn't look likely that we would.

The most exciting thing that happened in the week was an occasional Indian take-away. Although my GP assured me that I must be fit from all the running around, I knew I was piling on weight. I was also more and more reliant on my inhalers, which I kept under my pillow at night as I woke regularly in need of some form of breathing assistance. I quite literally just didn't have time to catch my breath!

We both knew that we couldn't keep up that sort of pace, but for the time being, there wasn't much we could do to change it. A friend from college visited one day and told me about a locum they had used in their practice. Getting a locum vet to work in a small practice in the utility room of a house with no vet nurse or reception staff was a very unlikely possibility, but Vanessa assured me that this girl would have no problems with it.

We decided to give it a go and booked the unfortunate Rowena for a Wednesday, thinking it would give us a mid-week break. By then Jack was also in play school, so we might potentially have a few hours of free time. Rowena called in the week before to look around the premises. I did show her the new building, which by then was plastered and beginning to look like a real surgery. If Rowena was shocked by the size of the existing premises, she didn't show it, although she had worked in many muti-vet purpose-built premises before now. She was happy to try a few days of 'sole charge' in its truest form.

When the 'day off' arrived, we left Rowena sitting having a cup of tea at the kitchen table because all the clients had refused to book for consultations as I would not be there. I was stunned by all the cases that, had I been there, would absolutely *have* to be seen immediately that could suddenly wait twenty-four hours. I was like a nervous mother, issuing lists of instructions, even though I would be in phone contact for the day.

Finally, we dropped the kids to school and then the difficulties started. What did 'normal' people do in their free time? It was a cold and drizzly November morning, so going for a walk wasn't very appealing. We had just had breakfast with the kids, so going for something to eat was out of the question. We couldn't go home because inevitably I would be caught by a client not wanting to see the locum. All our friends were at work on a Wednesday morning.

In the end, our day off turned into a trip to the local hardware store to pick the flooring and countertop covers for the reception in the surgery. After that we drank coffee, but always with the feeling that we should be doing something. We felt uneasy to be having a free moment and not doing something with it. We were almost relieved when it was time to collect the kids and go back to our normal routine. Once the kids were fed, Donal skulked back over to the shed while I took the kids to the local playground.

I was home by five that evening to check in with Rowena, who had managed admirably for the day. The clinic had been very quiet, she told me, although one lady did call in without an appointment with an injured pigeon. It seemed that the handful of vaccinations and the one coughing dog had not needed the assistance of a veterinary nurse or receptionist.

As I paid Rowena for the day she did admit she had encountered one problem she didn't know how to solve: 'Your farmer neighbour called in,' she told me, 'to deliver your box of vegetables and I wasn't sure whether you would want one head of cabbage or two?'

Rowena headed off to Australia not long after – I'm hoping not because of her couple of days at Clover Hill. If nothing else the couple of days off did make me realise that things would have to change.

🐾 🐾 🐾

As the building work approached completion, we were finally ready for painting. John, ever the perfectionist, insisted that each wall needed to be primed before the multiple coats were added. Despite trying to involve the kids in the building work as much as possible, we had to draw a line at the painting. Pink and purple wouldn't be the most appropriate colours for any of the clinical rooms although we did eventually give in with the addition of purple vet beds for any long-term patients (in addition to the more practical white which clearly showed up any urine leakage or bleeding or other forms of bodily fluid). Jack in contrast to the girls wanted to paint it all black.

We spent the May Bank Holiday weekend moving the contents of the crammed consulting room and portacabin into the spacious new purpose-built premises. It was hard to believe that the next day we would open the doors with a choice of rooms to work between. Although there were still lots of little things to be finalised, we were ready to open the doors and wondered who the first patient might be.

That Sunday morning, I took the kids to Mass, employing my usual tactic of arriving late so that hopefully I could contain them for the whole service. Within minutes, however, Fiona had managed to slip herself onto the back of the seat and fall backwards off it, clearly practising for her future as a gymnast. As I lifted her screaming body and ran out the door, with Jack and Molly close behind, I could feel the sympathetic gazes of the other parents. The screaming continued as we made our way out the church gates and up the road to where the car was parked. Then just as suddenly as it started, the screaming stopped.

'Birdie!' shouted Fiona, clearly now recovered. I looked to where she pointed and, sure enough, there was a tiny bird lying on the side of the road a few feet in front of us. Fiona has always had an affinity with birds of any type, and clearly this little injured avian had caught her eye, distracting her sufficiently from her own grievous injuries. I placed her down onto the footpath and she knelt beside me as I took a gentle hold of the feathered body. To my surprise it was as robin and apart from the fact that he was stunned, there seemed to be no other obvious injuries. His chest was plump and all wings and limbs were intact. Although I knew the likelihood of a wild bird surviving any sort of severe shock, we had to at least give him a chance.

As I drove back to the house, Fiona carefully holding the precious little body close to her fluffy jumper, it occurred to me that the robin was going to be our first patient. We made him a tiny nest in the cattery unit, thankful that it was empty for the moment, and connected the heat lamp. It took all of my persuasion to peel Fiona away from her new charge, reassuring her that he needed to be left in the dark to give him a chance to recover.

And recover he did. By the next morning, he was bright and chirpy and had clearly fed well from the food we had left. Our first patient was brought back to where we found him and he flew happily away.

I was sure it was a good omen, although Donal was slightly more cynical about the fact that the first 'client' had flown away without even offering to pay his bill!

CHAPTER 9

AN ELEMENT OF DOUBT

Now that we were finally up and running in the new building, and although there were a hundred and one minor details that needed to be attended to each day, it almost seemed like we could take a breath. Suddenly, just having three kids, a butcher's shop and a twenty-four/seven on-call veterinary practice seemed a breeze!

Now, of course, we had time for the element of doubt to arise. Until then, we had ploughed time, energy and money into what seemed like an endless project. We were so busy that we didn't even have time to consider the finances, or how we could make it viable – we just kept going, hoping that the energy of the whole job would keep us afloat. John was always the more conservative one. As a retired dairy farmer, he found it hard to believe that a purpose-built hospital facility for 'just cats and dogs' would be viable. I constantly slagged him about his lack of faith in me, but still he continued to count and record the number of cars that pulled around the house each day for the evening clinic while he was in the kitchen having a cup of tea.

When it came to equipping the clinic, he seemed appalled that I was replacing the old, second-hand kennels with state-of-the-art stainless-steel kennels. It seemed like only the other day, I had spent my mornings sanding down the old kennels, removing years of grime and paint, until the original metal was exposed and I could repaint the endless tiny panels of bars. The kennels had served us well in the portacabin, but in a brand new building they would have looked shabby, apart from being so time-consuming to keep clean to hospital standards.

It was a joy to watch the new kennels being unloaded from the articulated lorry that somehow made it up our country lane. The delivery man looked slightly puzzled until we drew back the original galvanised shed door so that he could walk through the (second-hand, but pristine-looking) glass doors into the building. It was a matter of hours before the shining new kennels were installed – two rows of four kennels for the dogs in one room, and in the next room (away from the dogs) three rows of three for the cats. Of course, within minutes the kids decided that they would make a perfect den for them along with our own dogs and assorted teddy bears. I couldn't even let John see the invoice for what they cost in case he passed out.

Despite his concern over the interior fittings, when it came to the actual building of the surgery it was he who insisted on everything being built to full house standards. It is probably the only veterinary practice in existence built to a higher standard than the actual house of the vet. Each room was fully insulated and soundproofed. The attic was sprayed with a fireproof insulation before the insulation material itself was laid down. The walls were plastered with a finish that felt like smooth marble and although the painting was left to me, it was with much supervision and numerous raised eyebrows when my efforts didn't match the quality of the work that went before it.

Terry, a carpenter friend of John's, was roped in for some of the woodwork. Despite Jack's concerns about Terry 'leaving his curls all over the floor', referring to the endless wood shavings as doors and frames were worked into shape, the end result was quite spectacular.

I did feel a stab of guilt when the three Polish men arrived to fit the white plastic wall covering in the theatre and kennel to enable a higher standard of hygiene and easier washing. They were quiet, but pleasant, and it was only after the first tea-break (which they insisted on having in their van) that one enquired what we were doing with the building. When I told him it was for a veterinary practice. He looked appalled.

'In Poland,' he said, 'we do not have hospital like this for the people.'

I did begin to wonder if maybe we had gone too far.

It was only years later, when the practice was well established that John finally stopped fretting over us even being able to earn a living out of it. He finally confessed that he had built the surgery to house standard so that if it didn't work out we could rent the house and live in the practice.

As the practice continued to expand over the years, there was no part of it that I regretted investing in. This was in stark contrast to all the large-animal equipment I had invested in shortly after qualifying, which still sits in a dusty corner of the shed.

But in the early days, there were many anxious days when the day's takings fell far short of what it actually cost to run the business.

With this in mind, I was delighted when a phone call came in one day from a new client. She had a litter of ten Labrador puppies and wanted them vaccinated. A job like this was just what I needed, until I realised that she wanted me to call out to her instead of bringing the puppies in. Going out on a call, a good forty-five minutes' drive away meant rescheduling kids, clinics and everything that went with it. But still, I wasn't in a position to turn the work away. I rang her back that evening, having arranged for Donal to get home early to take the kids, so I could do the call out and be back in time for the evening clinic.

It almost seemed like an afternoon off to be driving down the country lane through Aughrim and on past Tinahely. Being in sole charge of vaccinating puppies with no toddlers in tow was heaven! Feeling like life was just too good, I guilt-ily stopped off in The Stonecutters in Aughrim and ordered a takeaway coffee and scone, secure in the knowledge that I could eat the whole scone myself and that there was no risk of anyone spilling the coffee or scalding themselves with it. All too soon, I was pulling in the narrow gate that led to a quaint, comfortable country home to be greeted by Margaret and Edith, the two spinster sisters who had been born and reared there.

'Come on! Come on!' Margaret called out to me as soon as I had negotiated the narrow gateway, beckoning me to park beside the old Land Rover.

'Let me take your bag,' she insisted, almost grabbing the refrigerated bag containing the vaccines out of my hand as soon as I got out of the car.

'And I'll take your case,' insisted Edith, the other sister, clearly not wanting to outdone.

I suppressed a giggle as they reminded me of Molly and Fiona, although they were surely heading for almost seventy years of seniority. I paused on the doorstep to remove my boots and before they could hit the outdoor step Edith whipped them off me, placing them carefully inside the front door while Margaret continued on, linking me by my arm to lead me to a surprisingly spacious conservatory room at the back of the dwelling. Far from being for their own personal comfort, this space had been totally taken over by the family of black Labradors. One bewildered-looking mother and ten energetically crazy fluff balls greeted me with an exuberant, if somewhat deafening, enthusiasm.

Edith started bundling all the puppies, one and two at a time, outside the door, into the old-fashioned darkened hallway.

'Whatever are you doing, Edith?' questioned Margaret, although it was perfectly clear to see.

'Well, I thought if I put them out in the hallway, then we could let them in one at a time for their injections,' began Edith, clearly slightly miffed at Margaret's questioning.

'And wouldn't they destroy the carpet out there?' retorted Margaret, cutting her sister off with her tone of voice.

I busied myself filling the ten syringes with the vaccinations, not wanting to engage in what was becoming a heated battle of wits between the siblings.

'We'll keep them all here and then let them out into the hall one at a time after the vet is finished with them,' declared Margaret, ignoring her sister's valid protestation that they could equally well destroy the hall after the injection as before.

'Nonsense! They'll be quiet as lambs after their injections. Stop fussing, Edith!'

By the time I was ready, Lola, the mother, was flopped resignedly on the far rug, clearly glad of the break. Ten puppies is a big litter for a Labrador and as they were all very even in size, it was impossible to imagine how you could tell them apart. After the first few, as I examined teeth, eyes and ears, checked their hearts and lungs, felt for hernias of any kind, identified boys and girls and their respective anatomy and finally vaccinated each pup, the rest of the gang became bored and restless. As I finished dealing with each puppy, I handed it to Margaret, who handed it to Edith, who carefully placed it outside the door into the hallway, each time making a point of checking that they weren't doing damage in the hall. As the numbers remaining dwindled, the remaining few decided I was of no further entertainment to them and went back to harass the exhausted Lola. After a few minutes, she jumped up, spewing the remaining puppies in all directions and jumped up on the door to open it and let herself out.

'Lord, Edith, can you not carry out a simple task?' wailed Margaret as all the puppies ran back in to the room between the unfortunate Edith's legs. They scampered playfully around, joyful at being reunited with the pack, and clearly far from 'quiet as lambs' after their injections. There was a quick shuffle to ensure the pups I had dealt with were still separated from the ones remaining, and then we resumed the task.

Finally, I picked up the last remaining puppy. He was slightly subdued by being abandoned by all his play mates and he sat quietly as I made my way through his routine examination before reaching over to the tray to pick up the last remaining vaccination. As the tray was now full of all the empty vials and needles and syringes, I had to shuffle through them to find the remaining loaded syringe, knowing I had filled ten to start with. But much and all as I rooted through all the empty syringes, I couldn't find the remaining one. Carefully I re-counted the empty syringes; despite the last puppy remaining before me, I had clearly vaccinated ten already, meaning that one had been vaccinated twice while this little guy had had none. We all realised it at the same time and Edith was brave enough the be the first to speak out.

'One of the little beggars must have come back in when Lola went out.'

'Well that is entirely obvious, Edith,' declared Margaret. 'I don't suppose you have any ideas which one of the little beggars it might be?'

There was nothing for it but to confine the last remaining puppy in the crate while allowing his siblings back into the room and promise to call back later that day, as I had only carried the exact number of vaccinations with me.

Suddenly, what had seemed like an afternoon of freedom was not so appealing as I knew that by the time I made it home, I would have to go straight back to the clinic and come back later that evening.

The kids were not impressed to see me heading back out that evening and the drive had somehow lost its charm as I envisaged the hour-and-a-half journey to vaccinate one puppy.

By the time I made it back, the lone puppy was howling miserably at his prolonged confinement away from his buddies.

He was overwhelmed with enthusiasm as I took him out, didn't seem to notice the injection and then ran off delightedly to rejoin the gang. I quickly checked through the other pups in case whichever pup had received the double dose was showing any adverse effects, but they all seemed in good form.

Edith was nowhere to be seen. I suspect she had been berated for the incident, which was no more her fault than mine or Margaret's. Margaret had laid out a plate of sandwiches and small slices of cake which I ate enthusiastically as I filled out the ten vaccination certificates, not having eaten since the stolen coffee and scone much earlier in the day.

The puppies had been sold to people in the greater Wicklow area; a client of mine who was buying one had apparently recommended me to vaccinate them in the first place, and I was pleased to think that at least one of the pups would become a full-time patient of the practice. As I signed off on the vaccination certificates, I noted down the next vaccination due in three weeks' time for the new owners to bring the puppies to their own vets.

I had almost forgotten about my afternoon coffee trip when, three weeks later, I saw two new clients booked in for morning clinic, each with a Labrador puppy. I felt sure they must be two of the litter. Scrolling through the appointments list, I saw there were three more booked for that evening, and then another three the next morning. The remaining two pups came three days later with a family who had been away for the weekend and so delayed collecting their new charge.

I could well believe it when the new clients told me that

Edith, and especially Margaret, had been most particular about discharging the puppies and each new owner had been presently with a leaflet listing out the diet and general care and maintenance instruction along with a stern note that I was the veterinary surgeon to whom the pups were to be taken for follow-up care. No recommendation or suggestions – just an order! Furthermore, although this all happened well before the introduction of mandatory microchipping, the ladies had insisted that all of the puppies be microchipped in the new owner's name at the time of the second vaccination.

In hindsight, it was well worth the double drive to the out-skirts of Tinahely that day; it resulted in ten new patients to the practice, all of whose owners were suitably impressed by the new, purpose-built premises.

CHAPTER 10

TALES OF TABBY CATS

I t was New Year's Eve and we were well into life in the new practice. We had been invited to the neighbours' for the evening and although I was fairly sure that, whatever about the kids, Donal and I were not likely to last as long as ringing in the New Year, we were hopeful to get a few hours with the neighbours, many of whom we simply hadn't seen in the dark winter months unless they were unfortunate enough to need veterinary assistance. My optimism about not getting a call on the night that was in it should have been enough to warn me. It wasn't until I had the kids all fed and dressed and I was finally in the bath myself that the phone rang.

I knew by the tone of the unfamiliar voice that the plans for a relaxing evening were over.

'I could hear the weirdest yowling coming from the bush, but by the time I got back out with a torch it had stopped. I was about to go back in and then it started again and when I got in under the bush, I found this little cat, and her eyes were rolling and her legs were going in all directions. I have her in a box now, but I don't know what to do with her.'

As I got out of the bath and dried myself with one hand, still hanging onto the phone with the other and talking to the distressed stranger, I discovered that as far as she knew, the cat was not from the area, but from her description appeared to have been poisoned and was having what sounded like full-blown epileptic seizures. In fairness, she was very grateful when I told her to come up immediately and I regretted my initial feeling of frustration that while everyone else would be partying I would spend the night looking after a high-maintenance stray cat.

As Shauna lived no more than fifteen minutes away, I headed straight over to set up in preparation for my new patient.

It's funny how in veterinary practice, things often seem to run along a theme. Only a few weeks after moving into the new premises, Amanda the recently acquired practice nurse had booked in a routine cat neuter for a new client.

Unfortunately, when I arrived in to examine the new arrival prior to his surgery, I realised why he was called Twister. When I finally managed to coax him out of his cosy nest in the cat-carrier, I could see that apart from being a stunning, long-haired tabby, Twister had a distinctive head tilt and the pupil of one eye was significantly more dilated than the other. When I rang the owner to get a more detailed history, she told me that he had had 'a few' seizures, but as he was a wild cat that just came in the evening for food, she wasn't too sure of any further detail. When I told her that the anaesthetic for his surgery would carry significant risk and that working up and treating his condition could be costly, she reluctantly asked if I could put him to sleep.

I could almost feel the request coming, and I wondered if it was just me that got caught up with these 'hopeless cases'. I knew even before she asked that I couldn't euthanise this stunning and inquisitive-looking cat while he clearly, despite his issues, still had an interest in living.

Reluctantly, I offered for her to surrender the cat to us, knowing that now, not only would we incur the cost of his treatment, we'd also be left with another animal that we had little to no chance of rehoming.

I never regretted the decision, although Twister ended up staying only a short six months with us. Routine tests that we could carry out in-house gave no clues as to the cause of his condition. When he responded well to twice-daily anti-seizure medication, I reluctantly had to accept that it was not viable to refer him for tests that would cost more than all our patients put together would generate for the month. The anaesthetic went reasonably smoothly with a carefully tweaked anaesthetic regime for his neutering.

Once fully recovered from his surgery and stable with his medication, Twister became increasingly less impressed with his enforced confinement. He became our outdoor warrior –

fearlessly stalking through the woods behind the house and surgery all day, but always arriving back by dusk for his medication and a night in comfort. We became accustomed to his peculiar head carriage and his slightly exaggerated high-stepping walk as he prowled around his territory. Over the following months he never had a seizure that I knew of.

On the evening of a super full moon, Twister didn't appear and although I searched through the woods under the stunningly beautiful moonlight long after the kids had gone to bed, he was nowhere to be found. When a giant shooting star passed overhead, I knew that something had happened to Twister. Sure enough, two days later, Molly and Fiona came running into the house to say that they had been in Narnia (their name for the woods behind us) and found a dead cat. For some reason they didn't seem to realise that the dead cat was Twister. I followed them out and sure enough – although looking very wet and bedraggled and in their defence most unlike his former glory – there lay Twister, underneath a giant oak tree.

❋ ❋ ❋

When Shauna mentioned that this stray cat was a tabby and was also having seizures, I felt I owed it to Twister to take care of her.

In contrast to Twister, Titch, as she was named some weeks

after her arrival, was tiny. I had no idea if she was a wild cat or a much-loved pet, as she was so stunned and almost unconscious from the multiple seizures she had been having even in the car on her way up.

I rudely left Shauna at the front door and took the tiny quivering body straight down to the brightly lit treatments room, where due to her almost comatose condition, I easily was able to place the intravenous line, which would quite literally become her lifeline for the remainder of the night. I did eventually get up to the party, a five-minute walk up the road, twice for short intervals, but the remainder of the night was spent monitoring Titch and the concoction of medication that I was pumping into her to help control the aggressive seizures that were ravaging her tiny body. At the time I had no clear idea as to the cause of her seizures – her overall clinical condition didn't tie in with any of the more common intoxicants and although I couldn't rule out trauma, the few visible scratches on her head and back legs could have occurred during the violent seizures in the bushes.

Six hours into the New Year, Titch was finally stabilised. I wearily crept into bed, hoping to get an hour or two of actual sleep before the kids woke hopefully a little later than usual after their late-night party.

As Titch's seizures were now controlled, by the next evening she was recovered enough that I was able to remove her intravenous line, although this proved much more difficult than it had been to put it in in her comatose state. The frail, placid body turned into a hissing, spitting fireball as I struggled to peel off the sticky tape with one hand, while holding her thrashing body under my other arm. When I finally managed to remove the line, she shot back into the depths of the kennel, glaring villainously at me. I surveyed the parallel scratch marks down my arm as thanks for a night of intensive care treatment!

In fairness to her, Titch, once recovered from her needle fear became quite amicable again and would allow me to stroke her while feeding and cleaning her out, but in typical cat fashion, with even a hint of an injection or medical intervention, she turned into an angry tiger again. Within days, I discovered that her poor body weight was not a result of her medical condition, but simple hunger as she devoured everything I could put in front of her, including the dishes of cat food carefully laced with her medications. After a few days, she thought it normal that cat pouches and even dry food came complete with tiny pills and happily crunched through them without any fuss.

Although her seizures were well under control, I was still concerned about her slightly less-than-adequate neurological function. Whether the seizures had been from some form of trauma, or the severity of the seizures had resulted in some degree of brain damage, Titch seemed to have been left with limited vision, and her spatial awareness was questionable. As a result of this, she took great offence at being assisted into and out of her kennel each time and it was hard to assess her true personality as it took some weeks before she didn't look like she was being attacked by a giant monster every time we tried anything more than the most basic of handling. As food was most definitely her passion, she began to put on weight at an alarming rate, as we offered regular nibbles in an attempt to win her fragile confidence.

With her slow recovery and questionable temperament, I assumed that Titch was simply going to take over where Twister had left off in becoming the new resident. Almost two months after her arrival, her condition had improved to the extent that she could lead a happy, once somewhat sheltered life, within the right environment. The right environment came in the form of one of our vet students, who saw through the traumatised little creature and, at the end of her two-week work placement, arrived with a cat carrier. I was happy to discharge Titch to full-time veterinary care, leaving the empty kennel available for the next homeless crisis!

CHAPTER 11

I LOVE YOU!

It's often been observed that animals can resemble their owners either in looks or in personality. Over the years, I have certainly come across many such cases. In one instance, I laughed as a long-coated sandy coloured terrier cross arrived, wriggling impatiently in the mother's arms, followed by a trail of kids in descending order, all adorned with identical sandy-coloured locks. When I commented to the mother she assured me it was a total coincidence, but that I wasn't the first person to have noticed. Her biggest concern was that with advancing years, she might have to make regular trips to the hairdresser to keep up with them!

Oftentimes, short, squat men arrive with short, squat dogs while lithe, flowing women arrive accompanied by a dainty little whippet or the likes.

In terms of personality, oftentimes the temperaments match also and I have seen many apparently quiet, placid pups turn into deranged lunatics when in the company of crazy children. In complete reverse, a nervy, hyper dog adopted from an animal shelter can become an oasis of calm when integrated into a household of serene owners. Sometimes the personalities match from the start, but more often, the characteristics of the animals and their owners over time merge to meet each other.

Looks and personalities are not where the similarities end. It's always difficult when an obese pet comes in accompanied by an obese owner. It is the duty of a vet to advise the owner on the health risks and to recommend appropriate intervention, but it can be hard to do this in a way that does not seem judgemental towards the owner.

Other medical conditions can also be mimicked from owner to pet. One family in particular had three small children, all with varying degrees of allergy. Of course, as always, the dog was blamed. It always drives me crazy when medical advice is simply to get rid of the pet. When I was six, I was confirmed to suffer from allergy to pet hair and, of course, medical advice at the time was to get rid of the cat. But as the youngest of five, with four older siblings who had no interest in animals, I had fought long and hard to get that cat. Winky, the stunningly beautiful long-haired tabby with the intense green eyes, was the first true love of my life!

Luckily, when even at such a tender age I stoically informed my mother that if Winky went, I was going with her, she believed me and so we both stayed. As I pointed out to her at the time, I already had hard-set plans to become a vet, so I might as well get used to it. And I did, despite ongoing health issues. In time, my immune system did give up the battle, allowing me, many years later to fulfil my six-year-old self's vision.

Luckily, the allergic kids in question had an open-minded mother, who fully accepted that the benefits of dog ownership far outweighed the risks, and we worked together to find a way of minimising the allergic effect. Daisy, the dog, quickly adapted to her new regime, but then in time developed allergies herself. She was the classic 'big sister' dog to those small children, both in terms of her large size – she was some sort of mastiff cross – but also in her sheer presence in the kids' life. When her allergies developed, the family were fully convinced that she was just going out in sympathy with them. And it never once crossed my mind to tell the mother to get rid of the kids, even though, undoubtedly, their unending supply of treats was adding to her condition!

In my own case, having been born with dislocated hips, almost every animal I ever owned has had or developed some sort of hip issue. Of course, the fact that I have a particular attraction towards German shepherds doesn't help, but it certainly seems to me that when choosing our pets, it doesn't happen by accident!

❦ ❦ ❦

Nearing the end of a clinic, one beautifully bright June morning, I was reminded of this theory as I opened the consulting room door to admit my next clients.

Johan and Sylvia were new clients and had made the most of the Monday morning queue, waiting outside on the grassy lawn in front of the clinic with their new puppy. When I went out to call them, I was taken aback for a moment at the picture of the stunningly handsome couple, both tall and slender with dark features, looking like they had just stepped out of the latest edition of a celebrity magazine. They rested gracefully on the uneven grass, and I hoped that no previous patient had left a calling card, as the couple sat in pristine white – him in fashionable trousers and her in a flowing skirt.

Equally remarkable was their dog. While I have always admired German shepherds, as the years went by, due to intense overbreeding, the pups coming to the clinic have become increasingly poor looking. This pup was different. Straus, at a mere fourteen weeks old, was simply enormous. He sat regally between them, perfectly relaxed and confident despite the totally unfamiliar surroundings. The little terrier from my previous consultation, who barked furiously at him as she was hauled back into her owner's car, didn't seem to faze him in the least – it was almost as though she didn't exist. Straus, sat, alert and sure of himself, taking it all in through his big intelligent eyes. The threesome were really that perfect picture and I suddenly felt shabby-looking and became acutely conscious of my scrubs that, although spotlessly clean at the start of the clinic, had surely succumbed to a few stray dog hairs or dribbles or who knew what else? I resisted the urge to run back in and change and tidy myself up!

On a few occasions previously, living as we do in the picturesque garden of Ireland, travelling celebrities had arrived unannounced to the clinic, on holiday with their beloved pets. Unfortunately, due to the total occupation of my life between family and work, social media was not something that ever got a look in, so usually these clients went over my head, until they left the premises and one of the nurses informed me who they were. On one such occasion, I remember a slightly dishevelled-looking guy, whose name came up as a new client on the clinical records, coming in with what looked like a cross-breed pitbull. I wondered throughout the consultation whether he would pay or not, only to be informed by the nurses afterwards that he was in fact a star of some TV show and owned a holiday home in Wicklow and had indeed paid his bill in full.

It did cross my mind that the couple on the grass in front of me could be some sort of celebrities, and that maybe a few hidden cameras would be following in after them.

After a cursory brush down of my clothes, I called to them and ushered them into the clinic. Straus trotted along to heel as though he had never done anything else, and sat patiently on the weighing scales, before following the couple into the consulting room.

Johan introduced himself in flawless English, with only the slightest trace of a foreign accent that I couldn't quite place. As he shook hands with a firm grip, I couldn't help but notice the deep hazel eyes and his intense presence, and again I became slightly self-conscious.

'Allow me to introduce my wife, Sylvia, to you,' he began. 'Apologies from her, but she does not have good English. Yet,' he added teasingly looking at her. Sylvia smiled warmed at me with equally enchanting eyes.

'Well, I have absolutely no German, so you are way ahead of me,' I said to Sylvia, hoping she would get the gist of it and waiting while Johan translated. We both laughed as she understood. Despite the language barrier, she seemed to speak a million words with her eyes, and I felt sure we would have no problem understanding each other. Throughout the consultation, I was grateful for the presence of Straus, who, although equally stunning, at least allowed me feel more in control of the encounter and somewhat back in my comfort zone.

As I hauled his enormous body up onto the consulting table, I joked that before long he wouldn't fit on it at all. It felt futile carrying out a clinical exam on him, but I diligently checked his eyes and ears and teeth, before placing a stethoscope on his chest to hear his strong heartbeat. Although it is not possible to fully assess a German shepherd's hips until they are skeletally mature, his conformation was flawless and his already strongly muscled legs for a pup of his age were very reassuring. I wasn't surprised when, on questioning, it turned out that Straus had been imported from a German breeder.

Although now it is compulsory for dogs to be micro-chipped, back then there was no such legislation so I was delighted to see all of Straus' paper work in full order and with a correct microchip. His vaccinations had been started in Germany, so today's visit was simply to put him through a health check and administer his follow-up injections. He never flinched as I injected him, but graciously turned to lick me as I hoisted him down off the table – as perfectly assured and warm as his owners. For the duration of the consultation, every time I spoke, Johan would patiently translate each sentence to Sylvia who would always smile and nod back to me.

🦎 🦎 🦎

Straus became a regular visitor to the clinic after that. Thankfully never for any major health issues, but just for routine check-ups and weight monitoring. Everything was always perfectly in order. I couldn't imagine it would ever be any different. In time, I discovered that Johan was a life and fitness coach, and had set up his own business in the area, which was unsurprisingly thriving. Sylvia was a playschool teacher, which seemed to suit her perfectly with her warm, friendly manner, but she was trying to learn English before taking up work. I became used to our three-way consultations as Johan continued to translate each sentence to Sylvia.

Routine neutering is something I strongly advocate to all clients, for many health and social reasons, but in Straus's case I didn't suggest it to them as he matured. I know it is less common on the continent, and somehow there was always something so special about him and his behaviour was always impeccable that I couldn't suggest it.

Although they were probably one of the nicest couples we had as clients, and Straus was one of my favourite patients, their perfection was almost overwhelming at times. On days they were booked into the clinic, I found myself picking out a slightly more formal pair of jeans and making sure I brushed my hair at least! Despite my years of clinical experience, I always felt somewhat inept in their presence.

For as long as Straus came to me, both Johan and Sylvia always accompanied him, so I was surprised one day to see Sylvia on her own in the waiting room. I had never spoken directly to Sylvia without Johan to translate, so it was somewhat difficult to interpret as although she was studying English, her limited vocabulary did not, at the time, extend to veterinary issues. With a bit of miming and some educated guesswork, I figured out that Straus had vomited.

These days, far from lifting Straus onto the table, I sat down on the floor beside him. As always, he seemed in impeccable order, his now maturing coat was thick and glossy. On examination, nothing seemed amiss, apart from some very slight tenderness in his abdomen. With some dogs, it can be difficult to examine deep inside the abdomen as they are so tense, but with Straus it was difficult simply because he was so well-mannered that I knew that even if I was hurting him he wouldn't object or react in any way. I carefully watched his face for any signs of blinking or licking that would indicate discomfort as I probed his internal organs, but there was nothing. I was slightly apprehensive at not being able to procure a full history from Sylvia, but nothing overly concerned me about Straus' clinical examination. I indicated to Sylvia, as best I could, not to feed Straus for the rest of the day, just to allow him water, and to ring me the next morning if there was any change.

As always, she smiled warmly before leaving the clinic and I didn't expect to hear any more for the time being.

I was wrong. The minute I looked out the door the next morning and saw their foreign-registered Jeep waiting outside the gate. I knew there was something amiss. As the perfect clients, they had never shown up unannounced, always ringing ahead and graciously accepting whatever appointment was offered.

Despite having to get the kids to school, I let them in

straight away as Amanda hadn't yet arrived to open up.

One look in the boot of the Jeep confirmed my suspicion. Straus lay stretched out on a blanket, drooling, head hanging limply to one side. As I put my hands on him, he made brief eye contact with me, but then lost focus, his eyes appearing to sink back into his enormous head.

For the first time ever, Johan seemed agitated. Even his perfect English deteriorated slightly.

'He has been vomiting – every time I wake in the night. I give him water and he is vomiting again.'

'But when I saw him yesterday he was so bright!' I said, as much to myself.

'When did he get like this?' I asked, indicating the collapsed body in the back of the jeep.

'When we went to bed he was happy, like normal, but since maybe three in the morning, he does not want get up,' replied Johan, while tears slowly began to trickle down Sylvia's, for once unmade-up face.

I felt like berating him for not ringing me sooner. Providing a twenty-four/seven on-call service means that I always sleep with my phone beside me. I would have seen Straus hours ago if I had known he was like this, but now was not the time for that discussion.

Between us, we carried the great frame into the kennels and I explained how I would start him on intravenous fluid therapy immediately and take a blood sample, which I would run in our recently acquired in-house blood testing equipment to see if it would give us any clues as to the cause of his illness. As always, despite his strain, Johan relayed each sentence to Sylvia, almost as an automatic reflex. Her eyes brimmed up again as he relayed my guarded prognosis. Something that could cause such a drastic effect on such a strong dog was not good news.

For the first time ever, as I tried to reassure them that I would do everything possible to save Straus and at least to make him comfortable, I lost my usual feeling of inadequacy. As they both shook hands with me on leaving, for once, it felt like I was supporting them.

The day that followed was a blur. When Amanda arrived at nine, I eventually dropped the kids to school – their teacher being, by now, accustomed to the nature of my job. By then Straus was set up on fluids and I left Amanda running the blood tests that might give us some vital clues as to the cause of Straus' collapse. Having blood results so quickly would be Godsend as I feared that sending them away to a laboratory would be too late to help him. When the results came through, I was feeling slightly less grateful. Apart from being severely dehydrated, Straus' kidney and liver enzymes were sky high, indicating multiple organ failure. Although I couldn't be certain, the most likely cause was poisoning and the blood results mirrored my feeling of doom as I watched his once magnificent body, which seemed to have shrivelled overnight.

I broke the news to Johan over the phone – I could hear Sylvia in the background on the speaker-phone and listened patiently as he translated each sentence. Although deep down I felt it was hopeless, I told them we would treat him intensively over the morning, to see if he would respond. I offered referral to the emergency hospital in Dublin, but I was glad when they declined as, realistically, I felt it would just put all of them through more stress without any significant chance of offering a better outcome.

Despite all my feelings of inadequacy, Johan and Sylvia said they both trusted my judgement and the care we had taken of Straus until now, and they wanted him to stay with us, whatever the outcome. Amanda and I were quiet as we took a coffee break, neither of us wanting to acknowledge the reality that the outlook was fairly awful.

With the anti-emetic medication I had administered to Straus, his vomiting ceased, which at least gave him some relief. I sat with him whenever I could snatch a few minutes between patients, but he seemed to be far away, barely aware of my presence. I increased the fluid rate and the diuretics in an attempt to flush out his traumatised organs, adding intravenous steroids and a B-vitamin injection, frantically administering anything that might alleviate his condition, denying even to myself that he was dying in front of my eyes, whatever the cause.

I struggled to focus as I made my way through the morning's

routine neutering operations, thankful that there was nothing too challenging that required my full attention.

Over the morning, Straus neither improved nor disimproved, but just lay there as though fighting his own internal battle, oblivious to our struggles to save him.

I kept in touch with Johan and Sylvia over the day, each time ringing with no news, but knowing that they needed to feel they were keeping in touch. At lunch time, I suggested that they visit him after the evening clinic. Usually I discourage owners from visiting when their pets are hospitalised as although the animals can be really happy to see their owners, they are usually more upset when they leave, firstly because they have gone without them, and secondly as our pets are so intuitive to their owners' feelings that they are aware that there is something upsetting their owner even if they don't know what. In this case, however, I felt they needed to see how he was after a day of intensive treatment. Nothing was discussed, other than the fact that they should visit.

As the last client finally left, I felt like time was standing still. I checked Straus again before making my way through the routine chores and then locking up for the night. Amanda had left as I knew there was nothing more that we could do. I felt almost nauseous as I heard the familiar jeep engine pulling up outside.

Resisting the urge to go out and greet them, I sat with Straus for a few minutes before they finally came in. Despite the dark glasses that Sylvia wore, she was clearly crying, and Johan's face looked pale and drawn. There was little need for words. As the pair came over to the kennel, I pulled out some freshly laundered vet beds and placed them beside the kennel, providing a comfortable seat for them to sit with Straus. They didn't ask, and I didn't have to tell them, how he was doing. The once-magnificent dog was clearly in grave trouble. They knelt before him, reaching in and hugging him and whispering softly to him for quite some time. As always in these cases, I struggled with whether to go and leave them or to stay, but when I offered to give them some time alone, after quickly translating to Sylvia, they both emphatically declined.

'No, please no leave,' replied Sylvia, before turning back to Straus in tears.

I've no idea how long they stayed, but eventually Johan turned to me and in a barely audible voice said, 'I think but we have no option but to let him go?'

Tears brimmed in my eyes and I could only nod in agreement. My response did not needed to be translated. After a few moments, I pulled myself together enough to add, 'He hasn't responded at all to the treatment. Leaving him any longer will only allow him to suffer. If there was anything I could do to save him, I would do it,' I added, almost desperately. As always, as a veterinary surgeon, it is difficult not to feel that we have failed when an animal does not respond to years of college education and clinical experience.

Johan smiled back at me and then turned to Sylvia. I gave them a few more minutes and then gently explained how I would simply change the fluid in his drip to a concentrated anaesthetic and he would drift into a deep sleep before finally passing away. As he was so weak, there was no need to sedate him. I went to load some syringes from the carefully locked safe and as I came back into the room, they made space between them, graciously spreading out the vet beds, allowing me to kneel between them at Straus' side to administer the lethal injection. Just as I was about to open the valve on the giving set, out of the corner of my eye, I saw Johan turn towards me and then heard his deep voice say, 'I love you, my darling.' I stopped dead, thinking for a split second that Johan was talking to me instead of Sylvia.

My thoughts must have registered on my face, as I turned a deep shade of red, and in an instant we all realised the misunderstanding and spontaneously broke into shrieks of laughter. The tension which until that instant had been almost unbearable, was instantly shattered. We continued to laugh and then cry looking to each other and then back at Straus who despite his condition seemed almost to recognise the relief. It took us a few minutes and a few reams of tissues in what was the most bizarre last few minutes of Straus' life before we could all regain our composure. Straus gently slipped away as the blue liquid trickled slowly through his intravenous cannula.

I left them with him to say their final goodbyes. I sat wearily at the desk and dismally hit the RIP button on Straus' file, watching as his name disappeared from the client register and silently shed a few more tears of my own, somehow feeling a poor accomplice in this beautiful animal's premature demise.

I had sufficiently composed myself by the time they came out. Straus was to stay with us and be cremated, so at least we did not have to go through the process of carrying his enormous body out to the jeep. Both Sylvia and Johan thanked me and hugged me before they left. As Sylvia hugged me she whispered into my ear, 'And I *do* love you too, for all things you do for my Straus.' Tears streamed down both our faces as they walked out looking totally deflated as I gently closed the door behind them.

🗿 🗿 🗿

The impact of Straus' short life was so great that they simply couldn't bear to get another dog for some time afterwards. Although I bumped into them once in a petrol station, I missed them as clients.

Almost four years later, my heart skipped a beat as I saw their names on the morning consult list once more. 'Pippa', the new name read where once 'Straus' had been. Quickly I clicked into the clinical records and was stunned to see that Pippa was, far from a regal German shepherd, a terrier cross! I was fascinated to meet this new arrival and simply couldn't equate a terrier cross with Sylvia and Johan.

The clinic was busy that morning and it was some time before I got to satisfy my curiosity.

'They're waiting for you outside,' Amanda told me, so once more I made my way out to the grassy lawn and from a distance observed my new patient. The sight was very different from the previous time, where the magnificent Straus had seemed to match the stunning couple. This time a small, unruly-looking terrier hared around the front grass, followed by an exuberant toddler who shrieked with glee every time she made contact with the shaggy body. A transformed-looking Sylvia, in well-worn jeans and a loose ponytail, followed behind calling in, now-almost-perfect English, to the child and then laughing in mock despair as she failed miserably to catch the attention of either dog or child. Johan was not present, as Sylvia no longer required interpretation. For a few minutes, I watched the scene in total fascination as, although totally different, once again the dog seemed to perfectly match the owners.

CHAPTER 12

A NEW CAREER

They say that a change is as good as a rest, but in some cases, I'm not so sure. There is no doubt that having spent a year building the new practice, and the first couple of years working in what was a rapidly expanding small animal clinic, we could have done with a week in the sun, but in December 2008, a change was all that was on offer.

It was exactly ten days before Christmas when I was called out to a colicing horse late one evening. I was feeling slightly put out as it was a busy time of year for Donal and I had just got the kids to bed. We were planning to sit down with a glass of wine – more than likely the last one until after Christmas, as he would be working from early to late until whatever time everyone collected their hams on Christmas Eve.

Thankfully, by the time I got to the yard, Jill, the owner of the stiff old piebald gelding, looked to be in more distress than he did. As I drew up a dose of an anti-spasmodic injection, I felt confident that my services would not be further required.

'Just keep him walking if he's showing any signs of discomfort, and don't give him any feed until tomorrow,' I advised Jill as I headed back to the car.

It was bitterly cold, and the car had only started to warm up by the time I got home. Taking a bottle of wine, a box of crackers and some cheese, I went into the sitting room where Donal sat watching the news in front of the fire.

Unusually, he didn't ask how I got on with the horse, but remained engrossed in the news. In a world of my own, I busied myself cutting up the cheese and arranging slices on the crackers until the news ended.

'What do you think of that?' asked Donal as the ads came on.

'Sorry? Think of what?' I asked. 'I wasn't even watching it.'

On the nine o'clock news it had been announced that traces of dioxin, a carcinogenic substance, had been found in some samples of Irish pork. As a health and safety measure, all Irish pork was being withdrawn for sale – ten days before Christmas.

To the vast majority of people, this probably didn't seem a big deal. The news announcer had assured customers that any pork or bacon products could be returned to the shop of purchase for a full refund. However, to a fifth-generation pork butcher who spends from August to December carefully selecting and hand-curing the vast quantities of rashers and hams consumed by the population over the Christmas period, it was a very big problem.

Until recently, and for the previous five generations, Donal had used his own slaughterhouse, so tracing the meat to farm was simple. In our early years together, Friday nights had always starting by driving around a few small local pig farmers, where Donal would select the pigs for the next week. However, with ever-increasing legislation from the Department of Agriculture, the slaughter house had eventually become unviable for such a small number of pigs and so he had to source his meat from one of a handful of giant slaughterhouses where the pigs came from vast pig units instead of small local farms. Now it appeared that, having been forced to abandon the small local suppliers, the pork was contaminated and unfit for human consumption.

We sat in semi-stunned silence that evening, the bottle of wine left untouched, wondering about the implications of the announcement. The name Hick was synonymous with top-quality, hand-cured hams and rashers and it seemed that nobody could get through Christmas without a Hick's fry. Unfortunately, most people seemed to manage without it the rest of the year so that apart from the few loyal regulars the vast majority of Donal's business was done on Christmas week, which then carried the business though until the next year. To lose this crucial few weeks of Christmas trade could wipe out the entire family business.

Having spent some tedious months in food-safety lectures in my fourth and final year of college, I tried to reassure Donal that once the source of the contaminated pork had been confirmed, unless he was unlucky enough to have purchased from that particular supplier, he would be free to carry on.

By the following morning, several emergency websites had been updated by the Department, and now it was abundantly clear. All Irish pork and bacon was to be removed from sale and destroyed. No exceptions.

The next two days were a blur, with constant phone calls to and from health inspectors and department officials. Within hours, supermarket shelves carried only non-pork meats and for most people, life carried on as normal. But at a time when Donal should have been in the shop from six in the morning, boning and rolling the hams that he had been hand-curing for months, instead he was sitting at home in a daze. The staff (still known as 'the girls' although now in their fifties!) that had worked in the shop since their teens, before Donal had purchased it from his aunt had, with enormous regret and upset on Donal's part, to be made redundant as it seemed unlikely that the shop could carry on from the financial loss of a whole Christmas' trade.

Instead of cutting rashers and linking sausages, Donal spent the day on the phone to his accountants and solicitors, trying to figure out what to do next. His only visit to the shop over the following two days was to load the entire meat content of the shop into a skip and sign the appropriate department documents allowing everything to be destroyed. It seemed likely during that period that 'Hicks of Dalkey', the oldest business in the quaint coastal town, would be no more.

In the meantime, Molly, Fiona and Jack, blissful unaware of what was happening to their potential college fees, carried on in full preparation for Santa's arrival. The clinics were thankfully quiet as most people were busy organising themselves for the last few days of the Christmas rush.

I idly wondered what it would be like to have a Christmas with a husband not involved in the meat business. It seemed unimaginable.

But that was not to be, either. The solicitors' and accountants' phone calls had concluded that closing the business was going to be even more expensive than losing the entire Christmas stock. It seemed ironic that while the business was non-viable, the cost of closing it would involve re-mortgaging the house and more. There was no option but to carry on, but now with no stock to sell and no staff to sell it. We sat up late into the evening while a plan evolved.

Donal's parents, now well in their late seventies, were happy to be drafted into action. His father, the original Jack Hick, had never actually retired anyway, arriving into the shop at some stage every day for a few hours – whether to help or to check up on things, who knew? His mother, Betty, too, had worked a lifetime in their own shop, and was now more than happy to mind the kids and bake. One of 'the girls' also agreed to come back to work, but that still left less staff and more work at an already overwhelming time of year.

In my college years, I had usually gone straight from the last exam into the shop to help with the Christmas rush. I could cut rashers, although my sausage-linking skills were still in the experimental stages. I was also becoming a dab hand at cooking and preparing potato cakes, and had a few Christmas weeks' experience in hand-finishing cooked hams. Although I had never served behind the counter, I was the best offer at the time. It was a quiet time of year in a veterinary practice, but all the same, animals were still going to need emergency care. It was at that stage that Ralf, our neighbouring vet in Roundwood, stepped in.

'It's quiet,' he assured me. 'I can go down to your place and do a quick clinic during the day for anyone that needs to be seen. If anything is urgent when I am in my own practice, they can come up to me until you get home in the evening.'

It almost seemed too simple a solution.

The next morning, Sunday, I diverted the veterinary phones to Ralf, and dropped the kids, in their pyjamas, to Donal's parents where his father insisted on staying to supervise the feeding of a mountain of pancakes before he too joined us in the shop.

Fresh stock had been ordered from the pig units that had proved to be clear from the contaminated feed, and Donal and Jack Snr began the unenviable task of restocking the entire shop for the Christmas trade. Over the previous years, the demand for cooked hams had dramatically increased, so what had started as a kindly gesture for the local elderly parish priest, had evolved so that over half of the hams being sold were now sold cooked. It usually took the vast majority of the time over the last two days before Christmas to cook such a number of hams. It was painfully time-consuming, carefully dressing each ham with the fiddly little clove studs and glazing them with brown sugar before the last few minutes in a hot oven. With such an amount of raw preparation to be done, Donal decided that it simply would not be possible to do this in the short time available; for 2008 people would just have to cook their own hams. I began the thankless task of ringing the pages of orders to inform people that due to the pork crisis we would be unable to cook the hams, but to reassure them that we would still be able to supply the ham, although it would not be traditionally hand-cured as this was a process that took weeks to months.

The first few numbers rang out or went to voicemail and I was down to the third or fourth before I got an answer. Mrs Beacon was a lovely lady, Donal assured me.

'You're joking me,' came the terse reply after I had politely explained the situation.

'No, unfortunately not, Mrs Beacon. All our stock has been removed, and there is simply no way we can restock and cook the hams for such a large quantity of people.'

'Well, I'm not interested in other people. That's not my problem, but I am having eight people for Christmas and I have promised them Hick's ham,' she snapped back. 'I simply must have a cooked ham for Christmas!'

The next phone call was just as unsuccessful.

'I ordered that ham two months ago. I'm shocked with a shop with a reputation like yours. This an absolute disgrace.'

The third one sounded like she was having some sort of panic attack as she explained in short gasping breaths how she had booked to get her hair cut and meet her friend for lunch on Christmas Eve and how she simply couldn't figure out how she would even have time to collect the ham never mind cook it herself. At that she burst into tears and hung up.

I always liked my father's theory that we are all equally busy and stressed in our own mind, but just at different levels. As I looked down through the pages of orders I had to cancel, judging by the amount of time and effort that the first three cancellations had taken, I made a rapid decision.

'This isn't going to work,' I told Donal and his Dad. 'It would be quicker to come in and do the cooked orders myself than spend the next three days counselling everyone.'

🌿 🌿 🌿

The last week before Christmas was a blur. We were up before six each morning, delivering the kids to Granny and to the smell of hot pancakes. At some stage after tea, I would collect the kids and head home to do as brief an evening clinic as I could get away with. Poor Amanda was left with the unenviable job of deciding what needed my attention and what could wait. Friends, home for a few days before Christmas, later commented that they had rung me on my mobile to try to meet up for a chat, but that the phone was diverted to the office and they were greeted instead by 'the Rottweiler' as they called her! Meanwhile Donal and his father continued to work late into the evening, preparing the vast quantities of fresh sausage, rashers, pudding and stuffing that the customers would get through over Christmas week. We would meet at some stage late in the evening to grab a few hours' sleep before starting the whole process again.

The 'season of goodwill' has never meant much to me after that week serving behind the counter. Some customers were pleasant and would kindly enquire as to whether the pork crisis had put us out much. Others were incredulous. Why had we run out of stuffing? What has that got to do with contaminated pork? One helpfully suggested we should just sell chicken, lamb and beef although she walked out the door carrying her order in the 'J. HICK AND SONS PORK BUTCHERS' bag.

My limited skills were pushed to the extreme, and one lady did complain to Donal that the new woman on the till wasn't nearly as good as the girls.

The first day we reopened, about a third of the day was taken in giving refunds for pork purchased from the previous week.

We courteously handed back the money and apologised for any inconvenience.

'An inconvenience it surely is,' one woman assured me sternly. 'You've no idea how much this has put me out. I had friends coming over for a meal, and the recipe clearly stated that the four streaky rashers are essential to flavour the stew.'

I smiled weakly, trying to looking convincingly understanding, as I handed her back her couple of euro.

One caught me by surprise.

'I wasn't going to bother you looking for my money back for the pound of pork pieces I bought,' she told me. I thanked her graciously. 'But,' she continued. 'I did have a problem with them. You see I didn't want to eat them myself, but I didn't want to throw it out either so I fed it to the dog and he had the most terrible diarrhoea overnight. Do you think that the meat really was poisoned?'

Gently I questioned her as to whether she would usually feed 'Tiny' (her miniature terrier) a pound of pork pieces, conscious of the ever-growing queue.

'Oh, no,' she replied, 'he only ever gets his dry biscuits, but I thought it might be a little treat for him.'

I explained that maybe it was more due to the sudden change of diet and not the quality of the pork, and suggested she fast him for the next twenty-four hours and hoped that would solve the problem.

'Oh, thank you very much,' she replied, putting her purse

back into her handbag. 'You seem to know a bit about dogs yourself.'

It turned out that this wasn't the only implication of the pork crisis for the canine population. Mrs Jones wasn't the only one who thought that the contaminated pork would be a tasty treat for her dog. That evening I drove home with the kids once more in the pyjamas – the only clothing I had seen them wear all week. I was hoping for a quiet clinic when Ralf phoned me apologetically. 'That dog I saw for you this afternoon really feels like he has a blockage. He's been on fluids all afternoon, but we have our staff party tonight so I can't get back down to check him.'

With the kids dining on takeaway fish and chips in front of a DVD, I groaned as I palpated the dog's tender abdomen. Clearly, something solid, deep in his intestine, was causing the painful, ragged breathing, despite the heavy pain relief and anti spasm medication that Ralf had treated him with that afternoon. Amanda had set up the theatre just in case, but had long since gone home. I was grateful to my years of working without a nurse that I was comfortable taking on the role of anaesthetist, surgeon and nurse all at once. I worked silently, almost on automatic pilot, cautiously anaesthetising the little guy, who relaxed gratefully onto the surgical bed. Within minutes I was slicing through his midline, revealing bulging, gas-filled intestines. Following the gassy gut quickly led me to a sharp object within a loop of inflamed, small intestine. Thankfully, due to his rapid diagnosis, the gut appeared healthy so, clamping off both ends, I incised into the affected portion, to reveal a large fragment of sharp bone.

'Yeah, that's a piece of a pig's vertebrae,' confirmed Donal not long before midnight that night, when we were finally getting ready for bed. Thankfully Beanie made an uneventful recovery and was bright and perky when I left at six the next morning. I left the discharge notes ready for Amanda to pass on to the owner.

By 23 December, even the kids were getting weary of the pancakes-and-pyjamas routine.

In the life of a butcher, 23 December is the worst day of the year. All the customers are panicking and frazzled, as though only just realising that Christmas is around the corner and you know that you still have to deal with getting up the next morning. At least on Christmas Eve the end is in sight. Knowing it was going to be a long day, I had left a note for Amanda, asking her to put people off until eight that evening, hoping I could manage the few cases without an extra pair of hands. Luckily the majority of clients were grateful to be seen and glad of the few extra shopping hours. Of course I did manage to ruin yet another person's Christmas: Harvey, a cherubic Chihuahua with an aggressive streak worthy of a much larger dog always needed at least two people to restrain his tiny body to clip his toe nails, and they suddenly urgently needed clipping that day.

It was almost seven that evening by the time I got out of the shop. As I half-jogged the short distance to the church car park, I was mentally calculating how long it would take to get over to Granny's house to collect the kids and the promised lasagne and apple tart and get back to the clinic. I couldn't face another set of phone calls to reschedule people.

In the dark evening it took a few seconds to register that the large yellow piece of metal attached to my front wheel was a car clamp. I stared stupidly at it for a few minutes, willing it to disappear. I could have cried when the reality sank in. In fact, I think I did cry until I noticed a few other people passing me by, all dressed up as though looking forward to an evening out, throwing strange looks at me. By then the effect of the last ten days really began to sink in.

Desperately, I pleaded with myself not to fall apart for just one more day. I phoned the clampers' number and wearily recited my credit card numbers, at this stage resigning myself to adding another eighty euro to the massive overdraft that was eventually rolled into a five-year bank loan to fund this year's Christmas. When the clamper finally arrived, I smiled weakly at him, willing myself not to cry. I apologised if I had delayed him, reminding myself that he too, like the rest of us, was just doing a job.

'Well, that's what you get for spending the day up in Dublin shopping,' he replied smartly. I really – I mean really – felt like slapping him, but thankfully just didn't have the energy, so I sank into the car and wished him a Happy Christmas, hoping he would notice my tone of sarcasm.

It was late, very late, by the time I got home, saw the few (thankfully grateful and cheerful) clients, fed and bedded the horse and other animals for the night and got organised for the final morning of my career as an authentic pork-butcher's wife. The kids were well asleep by the time myself and Donal got to bed, exhausted but with a sense of relief that it was almost over.

Although Christmas Eve was usually an exciting time of year, this year, by the time the last ham was sold and the final wash up done, even the kids seemed subdued, any excitement turning into grumpiness as they too had been put out by the whole chaos of the lead up to the big day. Santa arrived by the skin of his teeth that year, cheering up the kids enormously as they bounced back into full action. But that morning as I almost dozed through Christmas Mass, I wondered how we had all got it so wrong. How it all could have turned into such madness and how people could delude themselves into believe that having a ham or a half pound of stuffing could make such a difference to what should have been the simple message of Christmas?

The Christmas Mass, which I normally enjoy, seemed totally meaningless that year as I looked around at everyone dressed up in all their finery. When my work phone buzzed, volume turned down, halfway through, I was grateful for an excuse to leave. Even though the dog in question didn't need to be seen, I walked home on my own, leaving Donal and the kids to follow me. I threw a chicken in the oven and prepared a few roast potatoes – the full extent of our Christmas dinner as neither of us had the heart for anything more. Then I sat and drank a cup of tea – the first fifteen minutes of rest I had managed in well over a week.

Thankfully, the excitement of the day and the exhaustion of the week meant that the kids went to bed early that night, and we followed closely behind them.

To my shame, it was Donal who was the first to think of the obvious point that everyone else had missed. 'Where,' he wondered, 'was the animal welfare in all of this?'

Prior to the massive changes in legislation over his years as a butcher, small farms had kept a small number of pigs, being fed local food and moving on to small local slaughterhouses. With the change to massive pig units, the pigs themselves had become just a number. The day after the entire Christmas stock had been loaded into a skip, word had come through that the factory Donal had purchased his meat from had been clear all along. Apart from the obvious waste of food, which could have fed vast communities of people in need, how many pigs had been needlessly slaughtered because of human corruption in sourcing cheap food supplies? For a nation of people who supposedly have animal welfare close to their hearts, there was little comment on the fact that so many thousands of pigs had been slaughtered because of human greed – at a time of supposed goodwill to all.

CHAPTER 13

DREAMS OF DONKEYS!

I dream a lot. Even as a child I dreamt a lot. Sometimes the dreams are hazy and disconnected; sometimes they are clear and logical. Sometimes the dreams are more clear and logical than the craziness of running a veterinary practice! When I first qualified as a vet, the dreams got madder especially when I started to do night calls – the bane of every vet's life. In the early days, I would lie awake every night that I was on duty so that when a call came in, it was almost a relief to just get up and get on with it. But as the novelty wore off and experience slowly kicked in, I began to develop the practice of 'automatic pilot' – I could speak to a client in an apparently coherent manner, dress, drive to the call, carry out whatever function was required in a relatively adequate manner and be back in bed without ever fully engaging myself.

It was a skill that came in very handy when the kids arrived – a big bonus for any parent. Sometimes I would wake up in the morning and it would take me a few moments to decide if the night's events had been a dream or had actually happened.

One such occasion arose after a particularly long week, where my sleep had been interrupted several times for a few nights in a row. The clients and kids had been particularly imaginative in ensuring that I never got a full night's sleep just in case I got used to it. Usually this was when the dreams became even more irrational and this night was no exception.

I couldn't even remember going to bed and was asleep within minutes which was very unusual for me. I've no idea what time of the night I slipped into my dream-state to one of those dreams that was at the same time totally illogical but very clear. In the dream the phone rang like an ambulance siren, but when I answered it, the call was from a client from one of the nearby housing estates who I saw on a reasonably regular basis with his two Jack Russells. However, this time it was the donkey that was in trouble. I'd say I could count on one hand the number of donkeys I treat each year, but who was I to argue with my dream-state logic as the client asked me to call out to a donkey in a housing estate who was apparently in great discomfort and frothing at the mouth.

Even in the middle of the day, taking directions is always somewhat challenging for me and I remember well that when I started in my first mixed-animal practice job, my biggest concern was not whether I would be able to manage to calve the cow, but simply finding the cow! On this occasion, I don't think even the modern joys of Google maps would have guided me to donkey in a housing estate.

Somehow in the typical randomness of dreams, I made my way to the housing estate, driving through back roads and wandering through a maze of houses before I was stopped by a man with a flashlight, guiding me to a corner house. Abandoning the warmth of the car, I followed the hooded stranger to a dimly lit back garden, which expanded into a significant larger space than was apparent from the front of the house. As the back garden became flooded in light, I looked in awe at a meticulously manicured garden, planted on either side with ornate bushes and neatly divided by a tiny pebble-lock path. My gaze followed the tiny pathway of the back of the garden, and there was a little thatched cottage, the dark straw roof in stark contrast to the brilliant white of the rough walls. A tiny red door was the only splash of colour. The top half was open, revealing the dimly lit interior of the quaint abode. Feeling somewhat like Dorothy in *The Wizard of Oz*, I cautiously peered in though the opened top half of the door, allowed my eyes to adjust to the light until I could focus quite clearly on a donkey standing in the corner behind an old-fashioned kitchen table and chairs. The dim light, I could see, was coming from the stove in the corner.

'How are you?' I asked the donkey, my voice sounding slightly eerie and out of place. I startled when the hooded man pushed past me and went inside.

I could feel the soft rubber of the earpiece of the stethoscope as I auscultated the donkey's slightly rounded tummy.

The eerie silence was broken by spasmodic gurgling in all four relevant sections of the gut, indicating that there was no obstruction or blockage. Magically producing a bottle and some needles and syringes from the large pocket of my waxed jacket, I drew up a reduced volume, to match the diminutive size of the donkey compared to my usual equine clients, and injected the liquid into the jugular vein running the length of his hairy neck. I looked around the small cottage and noticed with satisfaction that there was no feed available which might exacerbate the colic overnight. Leaving the cottage, I closed the half door gently behind me. 'Nice to meet you,' I called back the donkey behind me and felt slightly offended that he didn't reply. As I reversed my steps down the little pathway, I noticed the neatly trimmed bushes on either side that could well have been the cause of his night time indigestion.

My rumination was cut short by the sound of ambulance sirens blaring again, getting louder and louder with each tone. And then I woke, feeling the heavy weight of the duvet weighing me down as I tried to free my arm to knock off the alarm on my phone. As I checked the time, I realised with a start that I had obviously hit snooze a few times, as I was now a good twenty minutes later than I needed to be to get the kids up and off to school. I didn't have time to dwell on my gentleman donkey in his thatched cottage as I made scrambled eggs and packed lunches in record time.

On the way back from the playschool, I stopped in the local shop, picking the biggest of the still-warm, locally-made scones and within minutes was back in the kitchen, kettle boiling, thickly spreading the scone with butter and jam. I sat down with relief to enjoy a few stolen moments before going over to the clinic. Only when I was biting into the second half did I hear the text coming in on my phone. Feeling slightly irritated that my few moments were being interrupted, I waited until the last mouthful was swallowed and washed down with the dregs of the tea before I reluctantly brushed away the few crumbs and rinsed the tea cup. Only then did I check the phone to see what today had in store for me.

I sat back down and re-read the text a few times before it sank in. 'Thanks again for calling out to the donkey last night. He passed droppings about an hour after you left and looks right as rain now. Let me know what I owe you and I'll drop it in later today.'

As I said, sometimes my life is crazy and my dreams are so clear it becomes difficult to separate life from reality. That, combined with chronic exhaustion and an innate ability to take and follow directions, assess a clinical case and drive back home and get to bed without ever really waking up are probably typical patterns in the life of the few who attempt to combine on-call veterinary practice with three young children.

It was a few nights later, having a cup of tea with John, that it began to make a little more sense. John being John, knew the retired father of one of the last remaining thatchers who had been a friend of the owner of the donkey who worked in a local drugs company but did a bit of building work on the side. The little cottage was an old cow shed that had been left at the side of a field when the housing estate had built and the thatcher and the builder and taken upon themselves to reno-vate it into a traditional style cottage. I assume the donkey was only housed in it for my benefit that night, but still feel a little put out that he hadn't the decency to bid me good night after my efforts to help him through his ordeal.

❊ ❊ ❊

As I said, even when working in mixed practice, donkey calls were uncommon, and even more so when I was, supposedly, now treating only small animals so it was unusual to get a call to a donkey later that same week but this time I most defi-nitely wasn't dreaming.

Edward was a regular patient. Nobody could ever quite work out how old he was. I had visited him a few times before we worked out that myself and Edward had in fact first met many years previously in my student days. Every Christmas the Mansion House in Dublin hosts a 'live Christmas crib'. I can't remember if there was a live Mary and Joseph or a baby at all, but I well remember the wooden crib that was erected each year to house the donkey and sheep, and a random assortment of other animals that participated. Thousands of kids from Dublin and further afield remember the excitement of going to see these animals each year as one of the highlights of the Christmas season.

As veterinary students we were asked to volunteer to work shifts to supervise the animals and answer any questions the passers-by might have and – realistically – to protect the animals from the potentially excessive interest. I did it a few years in a row and well remembered the quiet old donkey who stood patiently in the corner, never over-engaging with his audience, always polite and never putting a hoof out of place.

🦌 🦌 🦌

It was many years later when I was called out by a neighbour who had been involved in renting animals to film companies to examine the donkey, who was slightly lame. Having dealt with the lameness, we sat down for a cup of tea and I began to tell Karen, the owner, about the student days looking after the crib animals. Her smile broadened into a wide grin before she eventually broke into a loud laugh.

'That,' she announced, 'was Edward.' It turned out she had taken over the care of Edward from his previous owner, the infamous Joe Gallagher, after he passed away. He was now living out his retirement, munching his way through a lush field in Ashford. It took me a while to be convinced that it was the same donkey, as Edward had been an old donkey when I first knew him many years earlier. After that we tried to ascertain his actual age, but we could never pin it down. Edward, it appeared, was timeless!

It reminded me of the time a local horse man had lent us a horse on long loan. Although standing at sixteen-two, Humphrey was quiet enough for not only myself, but also for the kids to sit up on, as Robo, the diminutive pony, had way more attitude than size. It was on Humphrey, that Fiona, at the age of five, had invented what became known as 'the giggling trot', as she would break into squeals of delighted giggling every time he broke into a trot.

Humphrey was retired from his hunting career, but still enjoyed leisurely hacks through the local woods and particularly enjoyed looking after the kids. His ability to look after his rider was remarkable and he seemed to sense when the kids (or more commonly myself) were veering to slip sideways; he would drop a shoulder or adjust himself in way to rebalance the most awkward of riders. When I asked his owner how old he was the reply was somewhat vague. One afternoon, as the kids were riding Humphrey around the front grass, an elderly lady and her grandchild were walking back with their dog, as our road was a common walking loop in the summer evenings.

'Oh!' she cried out in great delight. 'Is that Humphrey? He was the first horse I learned to ride.' I didn't dare ask her how many decades ago that was not wanting to offend either herself or Humphrey. Even though Humphrey enjoyed his retirement with us to a ripe old age, he still came nowhere near Edward the donkey's age. At one stage we worked out that he was well into his forties. At the time when all microchipping of equines, including donkeys, became compulsory, Karen asked me to make a passport for him and microchip him. Paper work was always my dreaded part of the day and although I did eventually insert his microchip one day when I was over with him, it as many months later before I finally got around to filling in the necessary documentation for her to pass on to the Horse Board for registration. A few days later I received a call from the same board and instantly wondered what I had filled in wrong or forgotten to fill in. 'There seems to be a problem with an application for a passport you have sent in to us,' came the efficient voice on the phone.

'Really?' I replied, trying to feign surprise.

'Yes, you have sent us an application for a donkey, and from the date of birth you have listed, that would make him in his mid-forties. There must be some sort of a mistake.'

'Ah, not at all,' I replied, relieved that for once it wasn't me that had messed up. 'That's Edward you're talking about. Sure he's probably older than I am. If there is a mistake,' I continued, 'it's probably that we've underestimated his age!'

Despite his years, Edward enjoyed remarkably good health apart from an intermittent skin condition and a bit of a tight back. Neither condition was in any way life threatening, so instead of waiting for a call, I would just drop in whenever I was passing to visit him. I nearly had the message saved on the phone. 'Is Edward at home', that I would send when I was on the way. His itchy skin always responded well to a mite injection, while his back responded well to a deep massage so that it became a habit that every time I called, he would be waiting, body quivering in anticipation as soon as he heard the car, for the lumbar muscle massage that would loosen out his left-hand side. As I pushed deep into the back muscles, his head would drop and his ears would flatten out horizontally so he almost looked like an old-fashioned bike with handlebars. His eyes would almost roll with relief as he felt the tight muscles release and he would stand with his lower lips twitching as though in a trance for a few minutes afterwards. To be honest there were a few late night call outs that responded so well to massage that I think half the time he feigned stiffness.

But the most recent call did concern me. I was in the bath late one night and when I got out I saw three missed calls and four texts from Karen. Although it seemed that Edward would live forever, I always dreaded the call that would surely come someday.

The phone picked up on the first ring.

'He's in a bad way,' Karen told me in subdued tones. 'He looked okay out in the field this afternoon. I only put him out for an hour or two because it's so cold. He had his rug and seemed happy enough when I stabled him this evening, but when I went over to lock up for the night, he hadn't touched his feed and he's lying down and won't get up.'

I didn't bother waste time replying, but got in the car and drove the few short miles to him. I was in the stable with him before I had had time to register what was going on. When I got to Edward, although he was lying down, he looked quite pleased to see me, his ears acknowledging my late night visit. I checked his gums, his heart rate and his gut – all seemed well. There were no fresh droppings in his stable, but I knew Karen was meticulous in picking them up and sure enough on questioning, she said that she had cleaned out a pile in his usual corner while waiting for me to arrive. I had to ask a few times before Edward shifted himself and stood up, but he was clearly able to stand and shuffled around the box reasonably well considering his age and the lateness of the cold winters night. Feeling bad, stripping him of his warm rug, I carefully felt along his back muscles and certainly those muscles on his left hand side were tight and he did his usual act of quivering and rolling his eye as I released them.

I was so caught up in the examination that I hadn't noticed Karen's ashen face as she stood silently by, as though expecting the worst.

'I can't honestly find anything wrong with him,' I said, breaking the silence.

We threw ideas back and forth for a few minutes as we watched him, but nothing really jumped out at me. Karen was apologetic, but I assured her I would rather call out to Edward on a hundred false alarms than have anything wrong with him.

We chatted for a few more minutes as I rugged him up again. He lay straight down, which was unusual, and despite my lack of clinical findings, we were both still concerned. Although I could find nothing wrong, he was clearly acting out of character and at his age the only certainty was that he couldn't last forever.

It was only on the way back out of his stable that I noticed something that I couldn't believe I had walked straight past on the way in – clearly my semi-dreamlike state and my concern for Edward had blinkered my focus. Edward's stable was part of an American-style barn. Years ago, Edward and his companions had been the stunt men, the business had evolved from renting animals for films to renting props for films. Part of the building was used for storing the props so you never knew what you would find when you walked in. If ever you were looking for some really random item that you had no idea where to source, all you had to do was ask Karen as she would disappear into the shed and invariably come back with it.

On this occasion, I gasped as I opened the door of the stable – in the dim light and almost walked into a real, life-sized coffin parked outside his stable door.

I deal with life and death in animals on a regular basis and I have no issues with any severity of illness in people, but I have a total aversion to dead people, ghosts, graveyard or anything of that nature. John often used to slag me when he would sense me getting anxious at the graveyard of a funeral saying, 'It's the live ones you want to watch, not the dead ones!'

But no matter how you want to rationalise it, parking a coffin outside the door an ancient donkey was just going too far. Karen was semi-amused as I berated her in no uncertain terms about poor Edward's trauma. Although I refused to help her move the offending article in the early hours of a dark night, not wanting to have nightmares for the rest of my life, she did promise to get it moved early the next morning as soon as the others were up.

She still thinks I was joking about it causing his apparent collapse, but I wasn't! The next morning, the coffin was moved to the neighbouring shed, and Edward got up and ate and went about his business as usual.

CHAPTER 14

PATIENT RELATIONS

I t's always good to be appreciated. Luckily, due to the nature of the job in veterinary medicine, our clients are generally grateful and appreciative for what we do, but as for the patients themselves, the response can be variable.

I can never understand why owners are surprised when their beloved pets are anxious or concerned coming into the clinic. Leaving the comforts of their own homes to go on an unfamiliar car journey is enough to render many pets, especially cats, nervous wrecks. In addition, they come into a waiting room full of the most bewildering array of smells and pheremones, which any self-respecting animal will pick up with way more accuracy than the more senseless owners.

When the first patient of the day is stressed or anxious or aggressive, the sense of that anxiety lingers for the day and the patients that follow are more difficult to reassure.

So I take absolutely no offense when my patients are reluctantly dragged through the door or have a quick piddle on the floor on the way in. At least they are honest and open about their feelings, unlike their human counterparts, who would probably do the same thing in the doctor or dentist's waiting room if socially acceptable norms didn't repress them from expressing their true emotions!

To be honest, I am more surprised that many of the patients, despite years of only ever experiencing such indignities as injections and emptying of anal glands, still bounce in enthusiastically every time.

Even more reassuring is the fact that most pets settle so well once admitted to the hospital facilities. Of course, we do our best, by keeping cats and dogs in separate rooms and making sure that the kennel is comfortable, in addition to the pheromone plug-ins that are constantly emitting calming vapour, but it is like they intuitively know that we are trying to help and once the overwrought owner has departed most animals are happy to surrender to our care. Often our most difficult patients in the consulting room become the easiest to deal with once hospitalised.

I remember one Christmas Eve, just when the last of the presents had been exchanged and the door closed, the phone ringing. Knowing that nobody rings after lunch on Christmas Eve for some trivial matter, I instantly knew the afternoon's plans were about to change.

Lizzie, one of my most obstreperous terrier clients, had been hit by a car. My first thought was that handling Lizzie on my own was going to be, at best, challenging. Until now, the most detailed view I ever had of her was of her teeth. Even the simplest procedure required us to begin by muzzling her, much to the embarrassment of her owner.

But on this occasion, my concerns were unfounded. Lizzie was collapsed when she arrived and barely conscious of my presence (which to her was usually so offensive). I admitted her at once, reassuring her distraught owner that I would update her as soon as I could stabilise Lizzie. I was quickly able to ascertain that although her pelvis was fractured, there appeared to be no other major internal injuries. By mid-afternoon the shock treatment, the heat lamp and the intravenous fluids that I had been able to set up while she was still stunned, were working wonders.

What was even more remarkable was the fact that whether due to the mildly hallucinogenic effect of the strong pain-killers, or from some life-altering experience on Lizzie's part, she now actually seemed to like me. As soon as she heard my voice, her tail started wagging, despite her continued discomfort. I hesitated before deciding to dispense with the muzzle and as I flushed her intravenous line, she gently licked me. Although I was still cautious I felt that warm feeling of satisfaction that I had made a difference and that Lizzie, with the typical intuition available only to animals, understood and was appreciative of my efforts. When Lizzie was discharged on Stephen's Day, even her owner was stunned by my new best friend's general demeanour.

Although I normally had to gear myself up for a visit from Lizzie, when I saw her appointment two weeks later for a check-up, I was delighted. As she was carried in the door (she was still being confined to allow her pelvis to heal) I could see that Lizzie was in great order. She was clearly loving the extra pampering that her injury required. Glad that we had finally come to a mutual understanding, I reached out to pet her shaggy head and only from years of developing lightning reflexes managed to avoid the teeth that reflexively aimed to sink into me! Although over the following few weeks, Lizzie made a complete recovery, she had decided that our brief friendship was clearly a delusion, and now we were back on more familiar territory.

※ ※ ※

Thankfully, some patients had no such issue with me. Hector was a larger-than-life Boxer cross who, from the first day we met, clearly adored me! It was only some months later that I met him down at the beach one afternoon and discovered that is was not only me but any human being that he adored as he ran from person to person as though each and every one of us was his long-lost best friend.

But still, it was good to be loved and, despite an episode of a painful stich-up and multiple wound dressings after an exuberant attempt to jump a barbed-wire fence, nothing diminished his undying affection and on each visit he greeted me with no trace of resentment for any previous treatments. Being a Boxer, he couldn't rest until he had licked every available inch of skin with the aid of his constant drool, which increased in volume with his excitement. There was just no way of avoiding the carwash-type greeting from Hector.

I hadn't seen him for a few months since his injury so I was delighted to hear his over-exuberant entry into the waiting room one morning.

As though he too had missed me, he was even more enthusiastic in his greeting, and I pulled out a wad of paper towel to dry my face as soon as I could pry myself away from him. Despite having a sinus infection at the time, I couldn't help but notice a particularly pungent odour from his mouth. I had a horrible feeling that the taste in my mouth was as a result of his getting just a little bit close and personal even for Hector.

'So what have you done to yourself this time?' I asked Hector as soon as I had dried my face.

'Oh, Gillian, you just won't believe what he's done this time,' answered Catherine. Hector was by now much more interested in the contents of the bin even though it had been emptied and disinfected since the previous clinic.

'You know the kids are back to school next week,' began Catherine, 'so we've been trying to make the most of the last few days and getting down to Brittas every morning for a walk.'

My mind began to wander, feeling slightly envious at the thoughts of a daily walk on the local beach that although only a fifteen-minute car drive away, seemed to be a distant memory.

'Well, for the past few days there was this dead dogfish at the far end, down near the rocks,' Catherine continued, as I pulled myself back from my reverie. 'So you know what he's like. I just put him on the lead in case he wanted to sniff at it or something.'

'Ah yes, that would be lovely, wouldn't it, Hector,' I replied, fondling his ears and remembering back to some of his more notable dietary indiscretions over the years.

'By this morning, the stink was horrendous and even he didn't seem remotely interested when we passed by, so on the way back I didn't bother to put him back on the lead.'

I could almost imagine the putrid smell of the week-old dog-fish rotting in the exceptionally warm late August heatwave.

'The kids were paddling in the water and I was watching them and before I knew it he ran back and just as I was trying to call him back, he swallowed the thing whole,' Catherine finished, almost gagging at the memory.

'Ah, Hector, you couldn't have, could you? Even you!' I asked him, subconsciously withdrawing my hands from him and remembering the enthusiastic welcome I had received. My hands and face seem to have developed a tingling rash where he had licked me, although Hector himself was clearly unperturbed by the whole event.

Catherine and I both agreed that it might be best to inject Hector with an emetic agent, forcing him to return the contents of his stomach. It was only after Catherine had left and as my sense of nausea was increasing that it occurred to me that our pristine kennels and white vet beds would soon be engulfed in the semi-digested remains of a well-rotted dogfish. Ignoring the queue, I quickly led the ever enthusiastic Hector out of the consulting room and, thankful that all the horses were out enjoying the sun, into one of the stables, full of a fresh, deep, straw bed.

Within minutes, Hector's face began to change as the injection took effect and soon he was forcibly ejecting the dogfish, which came out in one long piece followed quickly after by the remains of his pre-walk breakfast. Even Hector looked slightly stunned, as he dared to take a sniff at the offending object before quickly recoiling from the noxious smell. I stayed with him until he was recovered enough to have a drink and then led I him back to the comfort of the kennels, feeling sorry I couldn't offer him a toothbrush and some strong-tasting toothpaste.

That night, despite soaking in a hot bath with even my head submerged in the steaming soapy water while I held my breath as long as possible, I could still smell and almost taste the remains of the dogfish.

So although some grateful patients are a mixed blessing, I think the best ever love/hate relationship I have had was with a small terrier, aptly named Banjax.

Banjax first came to me late in life, but lived to such a ripe old age that we still had many years together. When he first came to us, he was in a bad way. He had been diagnosed with terminal liver failure by a large animal vet who understandably had neither the facilities or the time-commitment for such a tricky and intensive case. His diagnosis had been made solely on clinical grounds and, looking at the sickly form in front of me, I could only agree with the referring vet that he had both liver failure and a very guarded prognosis. His owners were understanding, but extremely anxious to do anything possible to save their only pet. It was late on a Friday night so I knew that the intensive therapy that would be required to give him any chance would be exhausting over a weekend without nurses, but as the couple were so keen to try anything I agreed to give it a go.

Banjax neither noticed nor cared as I clipped the hair from his spindly front limb, noting the yellowed skin as I placed the intravenous line and carefully tapped it in place, to allow me to administer medication and fluids as required over the weekend. His withered body was reeking of the smell of vomit and darkly stained with urine, despite the best efforts of his owners to keep him clean and comfortable since seeing the previous vet.

The blood results confirmed both my own and the other vet's suspicions that the little dog's liver was in dire trouble, but more usefully that it was most likely from an infection rather than a toxin exposure. I quickly added a potent antibiotic to his regime and knowing that the anti-nausea medication would have taken effect by now, was happy to leave him wrapped in an absorbent towel and well-padded by a few layers of vet beds. As I left, he looked both peaceful and comfortable in the soft glow of the heat lamp. I relayed the evening's events to the owners who were realistic about his prognosis, but grateful to at least give him the chance.

I waited until the kids were settled in bed before going over to check on my only charge so far for the weekend.

When I peeped through the small glass window in the kennels door, it looked as though Banjax hadn't stirred since I left him. He didn't move when I went in the door and opened his kennel to check that the bedding was still dry. Everything was perfect until I noticed that although the bandage looked undisturbed, the giving set had been neatly sliced through. Clearly, despite his weakened state, Banjax was not impressed with the unnecessary attachment and had simply bitten it off. As it was by now late, and judging by his clinical examination he was in a much better state of hydration than he had been on admission, I decided to let him rest in comfort for the remainder of the night and start again in the morning.

I got up early to check on him before the kids got up the next morning. I carried him out to the back passageway, where he drunkenly passed some deep orange urine before crumpling down on the blankets. At least he had stopped vomiting, but I was still reluctant to offer oral fluids or food so soon into his treatment. As soon as Amanda arrived at nine, I replaced the giving set and restarted the fluids, securely taping the line in place with multiple lengths of sticky tape. While the busy Saturday morning clinic went on, we regularly checked Banjax, but despite this, before long, the line was once again slashed. There was nothing for it but to employ a full time carer for Banjax. Molly was deeply engrossed in a book when I ran over to the house, but was still keen to come to look after this high-needs patient.

'Just keep an eye on him,' I instructed 'and don't let him bite at his line.'

With her eight years of life experience, including five in a veterinary practice, Molly was the perfect person to supervise the reluctant patient. I left her perched on the most comfortable office chair, having evicted Striper the grumpy office cat.

The next time I passed by, I could hear Molly's voice and peeped in to find her reading aloud to Banjax who, despite his grumpy old man disposition, seemed to be enjoying the story.

Banjax eventually made it home the following Monday, despite a poorly functioning liver, much brighter, eating and well on the way to making a full recovery. The owners were very appreciative of the care I had taken of him over the weekend, but I had to tell them that really it was Molly who did all the tedious work. They were clearly enthralled by the image of the eight-year-old girl reading stories in the clinical setting to their aged canine, and arrived up at the next visit with some beautiful books for her, along with the most amazing butter scones that Mary herself had made for us.

Although Banjax came from a long distance away, after his discharge, his owners asked if they could keep coming to us. As Banjax made a full recovery and regained his original form, I felt that the initial referring vet would be somewhat relieved as Banjax, despite his not quite six kilos of body mass, was at times as difficult to handle as any large animal.

Banjax had attitude and lots of it. It was only when he was well that I realised just how sick he had been to have allowed me to treat him and I was now amazed that pulling his line out was the worst he had got up to. Over his years that followed, Banjax suffered from a number of recurrent minor issues that nonetheless required regular treatment, necessitating regular visits to the clinic. His arrival was always heralded by a remarkably loud snarling from his small body and I was never in any doubt as to when he had arrived. He soon became known among the regular clients as 'the conscientious objector'. Once in the consulting room, he would keep up the snarling, which increased in decibels every time I touched him until I was finished, at which stage I would remove the muzzle, pop him down on the floor and he would docilely accept a treat from me as though he was the model patient. Banjax was all talk, but from outside the waiting room I'm sure it sounded like I was murdering him. In keeping with his character, Banjax was fussy about his treats, so that in the end his owner had to bring a supply to offer as he would look at me so disdainfully if I dared offer him something that was not to his liking.

As Banjax got older, the severity of his ailments became more challenging as he became increasingly debilitated.

One day, Mary arrived into the clinic unannounced and I could see by her face that something was wrong. We had already discussed that as Banjax had so many issues, should something serious happen to him he was no longer fit for any sort of surgery or major intervention, so I was worried. As she carried Banjax in, there wasn't a word out of him and in my anxiety I didn't even think to get his own personal muzzle, which was kept in a drawer with his treats. As I sat on the floor with Banjax, Mary told me how she had been washing up in the kitchen and heard a loud squeal from Banjax and when she came out his was lying flat on the floor and now seemed unable to move one of his front legs.

As we talked, Banjax picked himself and slowly shuffled over to me and placed his head and the affected leg on my lap looking up at me questioningly. For all the years of hardship he had given us, that one moment of trust and understanding between us melted me like no other in all my years of clinical practice. Banjax clearly understood that I was the person to help him and was asking me to do so. He allowed me to place him on my lap and examine him. Apart from a constant shaking in the limb and tight muscles I could feel no significant abnormality. I suggested to Mary that I would give him a strong painkiller and for her to take him home and keep him quiet and see how he responded.

Whatever had happen to Banjax, Mary rang the next day to say he had slept from the time he got home. Although he was slightly cautious on the leg the next morning, he was well on the way to recovery.

It was a few weeks before he next visited, this time with an infection in one of the many cysts and growths that had been appearing on his body in the previous few years. I was almost relieved to hear the snarling as her approached the waiting room. The old Banjax was back and as I gently drained the infection from the growth on his face, he roared and squealed at me, fully reassuring me that he was feeling well again.

※ ※ ※

As Banjax approached his late teens, although his attitude

never changed, he seemed to fade. It almost seemed that the effort of maintaining his status as 'conscientious objector' was becoming too much for him. His muzzle began to fray and although we kept up the old routine of offering his current favourite treat after removing the muzzle he might take or leave it.

I am glad that I myself was with Banjax when his last days came. We had discussed it many times and, although I offered to call out when the time came, Mary instead insisted that she would bring him up.

What is slightly strange is that I have absolutely no recollection of that day. I know it was shortly before Christmas. My clinical records outline how he had deteriorated and was neither eating nor drinking. The medications I used for his final visit are clearly recorded.

On the day before his demise, I clearly remember standing in the yard and having a discussion with a client as to how bitterly cold it was. She looked at me strangely and said that she didn't find it all that cold herself for the time of year. After the clinic, I got into a bath as hot as I could bear it and yet still the cold invaded me, so that even the inside of my head hurt. No matter how many hot water bottles I filled or how many duvets I pulled over myself, I just couldn't get warm and lay all night shaking with the cold while at the same time being vaguely aware that the sheets on which I lay were soaked in sweat.

I remember driving the kids to school, then ringing over to the surgery to ask the nurses to cancel all my appointments and crawling back into the sweat-soaked sheets.

Apparently Amanda rang me later that morning to say that Mary had rung to say that the time had come for Banjax to be put to sleep. Apparently I told them to book her in and to let me know when she arrived. I must have been a state when I arrived over. I assume I got dressed, but I doubt I wore my veterinary scrubs.

It was almost a week later, when I was back at work although still far from well, that I must have mentioned Banjax. Amanda looked strangely at me and gently reminded me that I had put him to sleep.

To this day I have no recollection of that last visit with Banjax or of his passing, but in a funny way I am glad I was there.

CHAPTER 15

EXOTICS

When Laura, a final-year veterinary student, rang to enquire about 'seeing practice' for a few weeks over the holiday, I was delighted. It's always interesting to have a veterinary student, as their enthusiasm can be infectious and although it takes longer to get everything done, in a nice way it reminds you of how far you have come yourself! It was only when she mentioned that her main interest was in what are referred to in veterinary medicine as 'exotics' that I became slightly anxious.

Far from being actually exotic, in veterinary terms, 'exotics' are classed as basically anything that, in small-animal practice, is not a cat or a dog. In my days in Ballyfermot with the Blue Cross, a pillowcase could be opened to reveal a five-foot python or a bucket could contain a dinner-plate size turtle, but due to the location of Clover Hill Veterinary Clinic, in the depths of rural Wicklow, approximately eight-five percent of our patients were dogs with the vast majority of the remainder being cats. The small remaining percentage was made up of the occasional rabbit or guinea pig, which I tried to avoid like the plague, not out of any aversion to them, but simply because I was violently allergic to them. As a child I was equally allergic to all animals, but despite the advice from the medical profession and my mother's despair, I persisted with animals at any opportunity until my immune system got used to it or maybe gave up on me. Unfortunately, as my contact with these furry 'exotics' was so limited, a simple toenail clip would leave me burning with a rash and hardly able to breathe for the remainder of the day.

Even less commonly seen than the 'small furries' was the wild-life – the occasional hedgehog or poisoned fox, the fledgling birds, which were despairingly hopeless, or the occasional call out to a deer – usually the result of a road traffic accident. Although I felt in many ways unqualified to care for these patients, I always enjoyed working with them; knowing I was their only option consoled me to some extent, and actually a reassuring number of them recovered and were eventually returned to the wild.

I did tell Laura that it was unlikely that she would see any exotics in her three-week stint, but by sheer luck, I did have one case that might be of interest to her. A few months previously, we had inherited a pair of chinchillas via the usual 'friend of a friend' scenario. The teenaged children had lost interest in them, and the parents had never had any, so Charlie and Mandy were looking for a home. It was unfortunate that Molly, Fiona and Jack were there when Donal mentioned it over the dinner table and even more unfortunate that one of their childhood favourite books had contained a full-colour picture of one of these silver-grey, captivatingly adorable creatures.

Of course we had to take them. It simply wasn't worth the argument and, in fairness, adding two chinchillas to our menagerie of existing dogs, cats, ponies, goats, ducks and hens wasn't going to make a huge amount of difference. What I did learn about keeping chinchillas is that, although not a great children's handling pet, they are, as far my experience went, relatively hypoallergenic as their dense, silky fur didn't seem to have any effect on either me of or the kids, who had inherited a, thankfully much milder, version of my allergies.

It seemed that Mandy and Charlie were content in their new home as although their previous owners had assured me that they had never had young despite being together for almost four years, about six months after arriving with us, I was woken by squeals of delight from Fiona who on waking, had handed the pair their customary breakfast of a dried apricot and when Mandy jumped out to take hers, a tiny grey fluff-ball tumbled out from under her. The fluff-ball was promptly christened Puffle, in honour of the ongoing Club Penguin craze. Mandy and even Charlie had everything under control and my intervention was not needed as Puffle got bigger and fluffier and, at an alarmingly rapid rate, started to resemble his parents.

Of course the problem then arose that as Puffle grew, keeping her with her father – I was reasonably confident that she was a female – was not going to be an option. Equally, much and all as Puffle became a family favourite, becoming incredibly tame by being handled by the kids (who in fairness to them had better animal-handling skills than most children of their age) at the same time, I didn't want an army of fluff-balls. So reluctantly I told myself that Charlie was going to have to be neutered. I have to admit I was slightly embarrassed, for all the times, I would silently raise my eyes to heaven as the clients came in with their pets' conditions already diagnosed by the powers of Doctor Google that I did have to scan the internet, in my defence, through some well-established veterinary professional websites, in relation to the correct procedure for anaesthetising and neutering a chinchilla.

So when Laura the vet student rang that day, I decided I could hold off the procedure for three weeks until her planned dates to carry out the surgery on the unwitting Charlie.

'My God, this is so amazing,' she declared on the first morning, as I brought her over to the house to visit our surgical patient. 'I've never even seen one of these. I can't believe I'm getting to hold one.'

Thankfully, I didn't have to put Charlie through the stress of a car journey, or admission and hospitalisation – I simply bundled him into my coat pocket to bring him over. I had already set up my anaesthetic chamber, having carefully bored a hole in one of Jack's old Lego boxes through which the inlet pipe delivered a mixture of oxygen and gaseous anaesthetic. Laura was as excited as the kids would have been if I had let them watch, but due to my complete lack of experience, I had decided against letting them be involved in the procedure.

'Look at his whiskers,' she enthused, despite my guidance to be absolutely quiet as we sat in the darkened room. In fairness his whiskers and nose were twitching dramatically as he sniffed the unfamiliar gas. I was almost holding my breath watching as Charlie gradually succumbed to the anaesthetic gas. Within minutes he was comfortably sleeping. Preparing the surgical site was more challenging than I had anticipated as, apart from his less-than-one-pound body weight, the hair was incredibly fine, but at the same time dense in a way that made it difficult to either clip or pluck. Eventually the site was prepared, with Charlie carefully swaddled in bubble wrap on a heated table to prevent his tiny body losing heat. Laura watched, enthralled, as I carefully palpated the surprisingly large scrotal sac and worked to manipulate the testicle from its normal resting place in the abdomen, through the inguinial canal, into the sac through which we would make our surgical incision to remove them.

The most difficult part was the stitch up due to the anatomical difference which meant that more internal sutures were needed to be placed than for a cat or dog, to prevent the intestine herniating through the canal. By the time I got to the last few skin sutures, I could sense that Laura was bursting to speak. Seeing that Charlie's breathing was calm and regular and with Amanda assuring me that the heart rate was regular, I offered to allow Laura to place the last couple of sutures.

'Oh my God, I absolutely can't believe you're letting me do this,' she exclaimed as she scrubbed and gloved under my direction.

The bursting enthusiasm dissolved slightly as I watched her hand shake as she held the tiny rat-tooth forceps and had to make a few attempts before grasping the edge of the remaining incision. Although I wouldn't usually allow a student to suture on their first day seeing practice, I knew that this may well be her first and last chance, perhaps for her entire career, to say she sutured a chinchilla!

I was beginning to regret my decision as she took several attempts with the tiny curved needle before finally managing to pass the razor-sharp pointed needle, threaded with the fine suture, material through the flimsy skin. After placing the two tiny suture, her hands were shaking even more but Charlie recovered uneventfully apart from taking a sneezing fit, his whiskers again twitched violently as he recovered in his little box, now inhaling pure oxygen to flush the anaesthetic gas from his system. By the time the kids came home from school, Charlie was happily back in his kingdom and eagerly grabbed the peanut treats as though nothing unusual had occurred. I was relieved that for the moment, I could honestly declare that

I had a hundred per cent success rate with chinchilla anaesthetics should a client ever ask!

Thrilled and all as Laura was to not only observe the surgery but to even play a part in it, her three-week stink was only going to get better. She was enthusiastic and diligent as we made our way through the week of itchy poodles and anal glands, lump removals and routine neutering and she was quick to learn so that I was able to allow her to do more as the week proceeded. By Friday she had neutered two tomcats on her own which, in fairness, is a much simpler procedure than with a chinchilla. Just after lunch on the Friday, I got a call from a Marc Ruddock – an unfamiliar name to me. When Amanda mentioned that he was ringing from the Eagle Trust, Laura nearly jumped off her seat with excitement. As Marc introduced himself I remembered that some months ago, a member of the public had brought in the body of a red kite that had been found at sea by the life boats. He was a wildlife warden and asked if I could radiograph the body to check if it had been shot or not. Although saddened by the lifeless body, I was happy to help, knowing that the radiographs that I had taken of my only other previous kite encounter, for the same reason, had provided enormous entertainment for my days of giving school talks.

Thankfully, unlike the first kite I had radiographed a few years previously, it seemed that this kite had not been shot although subsequent post-mortem examination and toxicology results showed that the bird had most likely been illegally poisoned and dumped at sea.

However, it seemed that from two isolated incidents of radiographing a kite my name had entered the radar of the Eagle Trust. Marc was now ringing to see if I could take in a red kite that has been found on the side of the road and brought to the attention of the wildlife warden.

Marc quickly talked me through some of the facts around the reintroduction programme, so by the time the bird arrived I was able to check his tags and weigh him. His limp body appeared almost lifeless and it was apparent that he was in deep shock. Within minutes, I had administered the vitamin K antidote in case of rodenticide poisoning, and had the bird carefully cocooned in a heated, dark space to allow him time to recover. His body weight and condition were excellent, there were no obvious fractures or lacerations and a quick radiograph showed no abnormalities – or none that were apparent to me on my now second attempt at interpreting a red kite radiograph!

It was only then that I rang Marc back to report on the case. Amanda and I did momentarily argue over whether the tag number had read 666 or 999 and with that discussion, Amanda immediately named him Damien, a name that stuck with him through the remainder of his lengthy life span!

Thankfully, Damien made an uneventful recovery over a three-day period. On the first day, while he was still barely conscious, I had to stomach-feed him with a gently warmed liquid solution, checking and rechecking that I was inserting the tiny tube in the correct place while supporting his slumped body between my own body and left arm. By the second day, he was bright enough that I could gently probe some diced meat into his crop a few times over the day and by the third day, I had trouble even picking him up as he was so lively and I had to wrap him in a large towel, carefully avoiding the large talons, knowing that if they grabbed hold of me that could do severe damage to my future surgical career! Damien ended up staying an extra few days until he was collected to go to the rehabilitation pens before being released back to the wild the following week. Although Marc invited me to come to release him, with the week that was in it, it just wasn't possible, but in the end I did get to see him as a couple of days later, as *The Irish Times* front page boasted a large picture captioned 'Damien, the Red Kite being released into the wild after making a full recovery at Clover Hill Veterinary Clinic'. I later heard that the local solicitor was slightly put out at how we had managed to get a free ad on the front page of a national newspaper!

In the nature of things coming in threes, Laura's luck was staying. In the third and final week of her time with us, after the chinchilla in week one, Damien in week two, week three was equally generous to her!

Bartje, a local neighbour's son arrived at the back door on his bike just around dusk one evening. I could see he had a bundle under his arms, which turned out to be a short-eared owl. Again I bowed to the knowledge of the internet to find out that these owls were quite uncommon in the country and only occasional sightings had been made in a few locations, including Wicklow. After slagging the neighbour that I would send him a large out-of-hours bill and expect payment in cash by the morning, I gratefully took the surprisingly feather-light body, which apart from the fact that it was motionless, appeared to have no obvious physical damage.

The owl, who was later christened Hedwig, had apparently flown at considerable speed into a glass patio window with the fading light and simply knocked himself out. Fiona, particularly, was enthralled by the owl and held the feathered body with a reverence that was humbling to watch. Reluctantly, I had to take him from her and place him into what was now becoming the bird unit, darkening the space and allowing him to recover with only the light from the heat lamp. When Laura arrived in the next day – for her last days with us – I casually mentioned that we had owl down the back and she roared laughing, assuming that I was winding her up.

Despite my warning that we would be unlikely to have any exotics during her stay with us, she went back to college with a case study of a chinchilla, a kite and an owl – all of whom made a complete recovery.

CHAPTER 16

THE HEROIC POSTMAN

T he relationship between dog and postman is well recognised. Almost every postman I know lives in fear of dogs and can spin lengthy yarns about the various canines they have to encounter on their daily rounds. If there is a postman training course, it should probably include a session on dog handling and behaviour as the most challenging part of the job! Although we have many postman clients who love their own dogs, even they are often clearly fearful coming into the waiting room of a full clinic – in fact they more commonly wait out in the car until we call them.

Of course from the dogs' point of view the relationship is perfectly understandable. There they are, doing a perfectly ordinary day's work, protecting house and home, either in sole charge of an empty house or, even more importantly, protecting their beloved owners, when an strangely uniformed, usually male, body invades the territory. This unusual unknown character is never greeted by the owners to come in for a cup of tea (apart from maybe in our house, where Molly's tea-making fetish ensured that the offer was always extended). The suspect then further unnerves the diligent dog by thrusting sheaves of paper, bearing not only his unwelcome scent, but also the scents of many other unfamiliar hands, into the letterbox and then without any acknowledgement, skulks off again, usually at speed. What self-respecting dog warrior would not be perturbed by this suspicious behaviour, day after day, without any logical explanation? As the pattern is repeated at a similar time every day the trusty canine builds up an anticipation of the event, growing in anxiety with each passing visit.

It's one of those situations where I can empathise with both parties. On one occasion, I was called to a house for the last visit to a little Jack Russell. Sophie, defying her gentle name, adored her owners, but was an absolute terror to Harry the local postman. I had heard reports from both the owners and from Harry as to her life-long mission to defeat his unwelcome invasions.

Harry himself was the owner of a great big slob of a Labrador and, as a genuine dog lover, was understanding of Sophie's phobia and had even showed me multiple puncture wounds on his ankle from when she had beaten him to the gate one day. He had never even mentioned the episode to Margaret and George, Sophie's elderly owners, as they were clearly besotted by their child-demon.

Harry simply took it in his stride and devised his own tricks and techniques to guide him safely to the letter box and back each morning, leaving Sophie, in Harry's words as 'at least a bit of protection on that lonely laneway'.

But in her later years, Sophie began to have seizures. Epilepsy is not uncommon in terriers, but it usually presents at a relatively young age and can be well managed. In Sophie's case, although for the first few weeks she responded well to the treatment, before long the seizures returned and with increasing aggression. I explained to Margaret and George that it was most likely that some sort of a brain lesion was causing the seizures and even if an MRI scan was a financial option, that a diagnosis would be unlikely to offer any realistic treatment at Sophie's age.

After one particularly bad night, the decision was made, so after the morning clinic, I made my way to their cottage to find them sitting outside in the sun with Sophie, clearly between seizures, on the front lawn. A half dose of sedation was enough to render Sophie oblivious to the sound of Harry's familiar green van crunching down the gravelled driveway. With tears in her eyes, Margaret commented that it was the first time ever that Sophie had failed to 'greet' the postman and that even the previous morning she had 'almost got a nip in'.

Harry was unaware of Sophie's medical condition, not knowing that the excitement of his daily visit often triggered a seizure within minutes of his departure and that I had tailored her medication to be at its peak level for his arrival.

Pulling up alongside us, he rolled down the window and recognising me sitting with the couple, roared out, 'I hope you're putting that divil to sleep!' I could see it in his eyes that before the words were out, understanding dawned and if he could have hauled them back again he would have. There was an awkward moment of silence before George graciously inclined that Sophie had indeed 'had her moments' over the past few years.

Harry muttered a brief 'I'm sorry for your troubles,' before moving on and slowly walked up the remaining laneway to carefully place the post in the letterbox. When he reversed back out the narrow lane, it was at a speed and delicacy that would have well befitted any funeral undertaker. With the untimely intrusion over, I proceeded to inject the intravenous anaesthetic that would result in Sophie breathing her last and was relieved to be pulling out of the drive myself after a sober cup of tea, at an equally reverential speed.

I think the unfortunate story went around postman circles for a long time, as even our own postman commented on it a week or so later.

My next postman versus dog encounter happened shortly afterwards and was, thankfully, a much more inspiring experience!

It was one of those days that was already so busy that I couldn't quite get my head around how I was going to get through it all when a neighbouring veterinary practice rang.

A dog had been admitted to the surgery that morning by the local postman, Frank Rennix, who had found him having a full-blown seizure in the owners' front garden. Clearly a dog lover, and unfazed by the sheer size of the thirty-five-kilo Boxer cross, Frank, abandoning all standard protocol and safety regulations, had scooped the fitting dog into the back of his van and rushed him to the nearest vet. Although he was able to supply the name and address of the house where the dog was found, as the owners were rarely at home, he had no further contact details.

The vet in question, focused initially on stabilising the patient who was discovered to have a sky-high temperature, whether it was as a result of the prolonged seizures or causing the seizures she was at that stage unsure. Over the course of the morning, intravenous fluids and anti-seizure medication brought the condition under control. The temperature dropped to normal levels, but with any reduction in the anaesthesia medication the characteristic spasmodic paddling of all four limbs promptly resumed, indicating the onset of full-blown seizure activity.

With the dog out of immediate danger, but still with a very grave prognosis, one of the nurses, filling in the hospital chart, scanned him for a microchip and was pleasantly surprised to find he was microchipped and registered to the name and address from which he had been brought by the postman. Until then, any attempts at getting a phone number had failed, so making contact with the owners was not possible. Although now with a phone number from the microchip register, the owners still could not be located as message after message was left unanswered. Decisions needed to be made as to the fate of the mysterious Brook, as he was identified by his microchip registration. Intensive and costly treatment would be required to simply keep him alive, without any guarantees as to his long-term outcome. In these cases, euthanasia is deemed to be the most realistic solution where no owner can be contacted. As the next line of enquiry, the persistent vet nurse decided to contact the veterinary practice where Brook had been micro-chipped and registered. When the phone rang in the office, I was elbow-deep in the abdomen of a dog who had swallowed a child's small rubber ball two days previously and although grateful that the ever-ravenous Labrador had not choked on the sizeable object, was unfortunately seeing my warning to the owner on the phone that night come to reality, that there were no guarantees that the ball would pass through without surgical intervention.

The neighbouring practice nurse passed Brook's details on to Amanda, who, after searching the client records, came into theatre to talk to me. I was surprised, as knowing I was deep in surgery, she would usually deal with such issues herself but when she told me the identity of the owner as per our client records I was stunned. The owner of the dying dog was my sister, Paula, or more correctly, my young niece.

The nurse was a little put out by the fact that the 'owner' had made no attempt to return the calls, but I didn't have time to explain that my sister was a consultant paediatric surgeon, working hours unknown to us mere mortals and probably involved in equally life-saving surgeries on people's children.

As soon as the rubber ball was retrieved and the Labrador left in Amanda's capable hands, I sent my sister a quick text saying that Brook was in the vet's, but I would collect him, and to ring me whenever she had a chance. I didn't realise the seriousness of his condition until I arrived at the neighbouring practice. I had the three kids loaded in the back of the car as they were on a mid-term break, all quite enthusiastic about going on a mission to collect Brook. Now that the dog had an owner, the vets had pre-emptively booked for him to go to the emergency clinic overnight as his condition would require continuous monitoring. The receptionist, who I had never met before, looked slightly sceptical as I trailed three excited children through the waiting room and out to the back kennels.

I was slightly taken aback as I saw Brook, normally an exuberant body of pure energy and enthusiasm, lying lifeless in the bottom kennel, apart from the subtle sporadic twitching of his limbs, indicating that his body was still battling the unknown cause of his condition. The kids were equally taken aback and hung back in shock; they had obviously been expecting the

Brook they knew and loved, who'd flattened them on numerous occasions with his joyful welcomes.

Fiona, always the sensitive one, began to cry, while Jack busied himself examining the nuts and bolts on the drip stand.

For any other client, I simply couldn't, legally or any other way, transport an anaesthetised, seriously-ill animal in the boot of my car, on my own dog's bed with three children in the back seat, without so much as informing the owner, never mind getting consent, but in the case of your sister, rules can be bent. Despite her slight anxiety, the nurse on duty allowed me to top up his anaesthetic with a slightly more long-acting intravenous medication, watching cautiously as I drew up a dose that would hopefully keep him stable for the relatively short journey home. I drew up an extra dose in case of unexpected delays on the way home.

Trying not to think of my many discussions with my sister of the team of anaesthetists that would monitor the patient while she operated and the post-operative intensive care monitoring, I bundled the sleeping Brook into the boot of the car while Molly, with the efficiency of the eldest sibling, busied herself buckling Jack and Fiona into their seats, sensing the urgency on hand.

I stayed a hair's breadth below the speed limit all the way home, listening, over the kids' excited squabbling as to how who would mind Brook, for his breathing, which was irregular and harsh. After a few minutes of dispute, Molly as the undisputed eldest child, proclaimed that I was the vet, but she would be the main minder as Paula was her godmother so, by that argument, Brook would be her godbrother. Fiona acquiesced, but not without offering a favourite unicorn to accompany him in the kennels.

By the time we made it back to the surgery, Brook's breathing was becoming lighter and the limb twitching was getting stronger. I topped up his medication in the boot of the car, not wanting to move him while he was unstable. Before long, we had him settled in a kennel and stable once more and I couldn't help wondering if at any level of his consciousness he was aware of the drama of the day unfolding? Misty the Labrador was doing well and sitting up, interested in the whole proceedings, as we drew bloods from Brook to see if they would give us any indications to the cause of his dramatic illness.

As Donal was now back home, I was able to focus on the evening clinic, without the aid of my junior assistants. While Amanda monitored Brook, I worked my way through the long waiting list, at one stage absently-mindedly noticing that it was quite some time since I had eaten. It was after eight when I had finished, and noticed a missed call on the phone from my brother-in-law. As an ex-agricultural scientist, he was ostensibly unperturbed by the whole event and promised to make contact with the postman, without whose intervention he would have returned with the kids after their hurling match to find a dead dog on the lawn.

The blood results had indicated that the most likely cause was poisoning although without more significant and costly analysis it would be difficult to prove. Both his liver and kidneys were struggling and I had to be realistic about his long-term prognosis.

'Even if he does pull though, Jim, there might be too much damage to his organs. And there is only so long we can keep him safely anaesthetised.'

As a husband to a surgeon there was little I had to explain to him, apart from the difference in intensive care in a children's referral hospital and a one-vet veterinary practice.

I did, of course, offer to send him to the emergency clinic but was unsurprised when he was adamant that Brook stay where he was.

By three o'clock that morning, I was beginning to regret his faith in me. Brook was still requiring deep anaesthesia to control the seizures and at that hour my brain was screaming resistance to trying to work out a fluid rate to maintain his kidney function while flushing out his toxic liver. Although I only had to hop a fence in my pyjamas to go from the house to the surgery, it seemed a long night. Jack decided to go out in sympathy with my disturbed night and woke frequently, syncing his times with the times when Brook was stable. At one stage I made myself a mug of hot chocolate and wearily munched on a handful of chocolate digestives, hoping they would give a bit of false energy to get me through the night. It was the early hours of the morning when I noticed a text from my sister who was clearly having a night like mine. Despite the hour, I texted her back, without being able to give any positive reassurance, knowing that she was as likely to be up at that hour as any other. The reply came almost instantly. She was even more realistic than me, knowing well the gravity of the situation.

By morning, Brook was neither better nor worse, still twitching slightly, but at least his temperature was stable and his urine output was copious – liberally soaking me every time I moved him! At least for the day time, I had Amanda and our new trainee nurse to take over some of the monitoring and I got to rest for a few hours in the afternoon, semi-slumbering on the couch in front of the TV with the kids.

By night time, Brook was frustratingly the same – perfectly comfortable, but showing absolutely no signs of improvement. I almost began to wish that something would change, either way. Despite Jim and Paula's assurance that their kids were fine, I was sure they were struggling, not knowing whether their larger-than-life buddy was going to make it or not.

I had to make a decision. I knew from experience that I could do one night of up-all-night and still just about function the next day, but after the second night I simply wouldn't be in a fit state to work or be responsible for three children. Ignoring all normal protocol, I packed a few boxes, and, with Donal's help, hauled all the equipment that I would need to keep Brook stable for the night, over to the kitchen. The kids were delighted, preparing a thick bed of duvets and covering it with plastic and towels. I placed my drugs and syringes high up in a press, well out of reach of any inquisitive hands.

So that second night Brook stayed on the kitchen floor while I managing to top up his medications and monitoring without the journey over and back to the surgery. I had, on a few occasions, spent some or all of the night in the kennels with a patient requiring intensive monitoring, prior to the setting up of the Dublin emergency clinic, but at least with Brook in the kitchen I was still close to kids and could enjoy the comfort of my own bed even if for very short periods.

By this stage, all efforts at keeping monitoring records – often the most tedious part of a time-intensive case – had been dispensed with (thankfully a sister cannot really be regarded as a client and it was unlikely she would sue me if things went wrong). And really there was no change to record. Brook stayed stable but with as little sign of improvement as of deterioration. Each time I tried to reduce the dose of anaesthetic, the seizure activity immediately began to increase.

The phone calls to Jim or my sister, whichever was available, became increasingly futile as I relayed the same message each time. It was Paula who brought up the possibility of putting him to sleep. Apparently, the anaesthetists in the children's hospital were intrigued by the daily drama and fascinated with how a dog in a humble vet's kitchen could still be going, two days later.

By the third morning, as I tried to organise breakfast for the kids while Brook lay slumbering, attached to all the medical paraphernalia, it was Fiona who sat chatting to the patient. As I served up the hurried breakfast, I was intrigued by her continuous giggling as she sat talking to him.

'He's wagging his tail at me,' she announced.

I didn't bother to explain that his wagging tail was nothing more than twitching. Who was I to burst the bubble of a five-year-old? Amanda helped to carry Brook and all his equipment back to the surgery the next morning. Before moving him, I again increased the medication slightly, fearing that the movement could trigger a major seizure, which at this stage would make the efforts of the past forty-eight hours futile.

Before the evening clinic started, we repeated the blood tests, and although there was slight improvement in his kidney function, his liver was still struggling.

Wednesday was our half day at work, dating back to the days when I would close early to go my Blue Cross clinic in Ballyfermot on a Wednesday evening. At lunch-time, we had to reverse the journey of carrying Brook back to the kitchen to his designated hospital bed in front of the stove.

Fiona sat, arranging the increasing supply of teddy bears around his bed, thankfully not noticing the ones that went missing in the night after he had piddled on them.

I washed the dishes in slow-motion, wondering how long

I could put off ringing my sister; we had agreed that three days would be, as far as we would let it go without any signs of improvement before having to make the decision to push the anaesthetic past the dose of no return. I knew that the amount and duration of the medication in his system was dangerously close to, if not beyond, toxic levels. In the absence of the required level of intensive care monitoring equipment, it was reaching the stage where I was potentially doing more harm than good.

My internal struggle was broken by the sound of Fiona's not unfamiliar giggling.

'Stop tickling me,' she squealed. I turned absent mindedly to prevent the squabbling only to see that she was lying alongside Brook and he *was* tickling her – his tail lazily wagging up and down across her head as it rested on his broad back. Quickly I glanced to the kitchen clock to see that yes, he had been due his next top up some fifteen minutes previously. Each time, I would wait for his depth of anaesthesia to drop and not until the tell-tale paddling limbs resumed would I add more anaesthetic via a port to his intravenous line.

But this time, although the heart rate had increased slightly, there was no limb paddling, only an intermittent wagging of the tail every time Fiona giggled. As I had long giving up on the charts, I could not fill in the response to *external* stimuli section with 'wagged tail in response to child giggling'! Which was just as well as it would be never be approved if the case ever did get to being published in some fancy scientific journal. But yes, there it was again, the definite tail wag with each episode of giggling.

Fiona, delighted with herself for 'fixing Brook', was slightly put out when I had to relieve her of her duties, as allowing Brook to gradually come out of his enforced sleep could be slightly dangerous as his behaviour could be somewhat unpredictable and he could even be aggressive.

The next positive reflex I got was about two hours later, when the more continuous tail-wagging episodes progressed to a quick lick of my nose as I peered in the back of his eyes with the ophthalmoscope trying to ascertain his eye reflexes.

I tried to ring Paula a couple of times that evening and when she didn't answer, I assumed she was avoiding the bad news. When I finally got hold of her, I was able to report that there was some progress, but although things were looking more positive, I still couldn't guarantee that Brook would return to normal function.

But return to normal function he did! Although he stayed with us for almost a week, reluctantly giving up his stove-side private room to be downgraded to a general public hospital ward, by the following week he was fit to go home although he had lost a massive amount of weight and his blood results were still of concern. Six months later he finally got the all clear, when the last blood result returned to normal after a special liver diet that allowed his liver to rest and, as is often the case in a young and otherwise healthy dog, rebuild its own normal function.

We never did find out for sure the cause of Brook's poisoning and I never did get to write up a scientific case report for the *Vet Journal* due to the absence of intensive care records.

And Frank, the postman in question, became a bit of a local hero – at least in the eyes of the kids who got their larger-than-life buddy back in one piece.

CHAPTER 17

AN INTIMATE
RELATIONSHIP!

I t seemed that the red kite reintroduction programme that I'd learned about from Marc was succeeding as, at first occasionally, but then with increasing frequency, I would see red kites circling and hear their distinctive cry in the woods behind us. When we first moved to the area, there was a nest of buzzards that we would see while out walking in the woods and they seemed to become accustomed to us as we passed, initially with buggies and back packs full of kids and, as the years went by, with our more adventurous explorers. The trees where they nested were tall, and they would sit and watch us and occasionally fly over us as though marking their territory.

It was some months after Damien's visit to us that I first saw a kite circling in the woods behind us. Over the years, as the kite population grew, the buzzards kept to one side of the woods while the kites, in general, kept to the lower side. In years to come, as the populations continued to expand, it seemed that a road divided their territory. I would sometimes see a kite perched high up in a tree on one side of the road, with a buzzard on his perch on the opposite side with a distance of no more than twenty or so feet separating them. All in all, it appeared to be a very amicable neighbourhood!

It was probably well over a year after Damien's visit that I woke one Monday morning to see the local wildlife warden's van pulling into the driveway. I had spent the weekend sick in bed and, as Donal didn't open the shop on a Monday, he had dropped the kids to school and I had been hoping to get an extra hour in bed before going over to the clinic at ten. After a few minutes of bracing myself, my curiosity got the better of me. I slowly dressed and opened the gate instead of climbing it as I usually did, to go over to the surgery.

I didn't know the new wildlife warden, but the box looked interestingly large and, sure enough, he pulled back the straw to reveal another red kite. Rough and all as I felt, the unfortunate kite looked a lot worse. He had been found in a ditch under some electricity pylons, and the assumption was that he had flown into some wires at speed. Despite my previous success with Damien, this guy looked fairly hopeless, but I went through the motions of weighing him, checking his tag number, injecting him with antidote, radiographing his body and full wingspan and then bundling him into what was now officially the bird unit under a heat lamp.

Marc rang later that morning and I told him that it was

unlikely that the bird would make it. He was a good weight and – after getting through the wet and tousled feathers – I'd found that his condition had been good before the accident, but now he was severely shocked and, in addition, had a nasty, open-fractured wing. The harsh reality of working with wildlife is that if they cannot return to one hundred percent health, where they will be able to hunt and feed themselves, it is not compassionate to keep them alive. A kite with an open-fractured wing, with the bone protruding through wet and dirty feathers has a very poor chance of returning to perfect flight. As we chatted, we were both obviously pondering the options, but neither of us could make the call to simply euthanise him.

Ciaran, as he later became known, ended up spending almost six months with us, as he recovered sufficiently in the first few days to make it through an anaesthetic for the surgery to repair his wing. The wing, in the end, healed around the tiny pin that I had had to adapt to drill into the hollow wing-bone. However, due to the severity of the soft-tissue damage, and the complications of infection, he developed muscle adhesions that did not allow him to return to perfect, hunting, survival flight. The level of care that he required and received, especially in the early days when he had to be tube-fed on a regular basis before gradually progressing to crop feeding, meant that he became tame to the extent that he eventually ended up becoming a permanent, fully-engaged, and cheeky resident in a falconry.

If I had known at the start how much work would be involved in his recovery, I might have hesitated. I didn't dare ask Amanda to add care of a comatose kite to her already busy daily workload and was happy to take full responsibility for him myself. For the six months he stayed with us, checking the in-patients and locking up at night, usually around half-ten or eleven at night, after the kids were all in bed asleep would be his time. Of course, his general care, treatment and feeding went on throughout the day, but with other patients to care for, along with their owners and with all that was going on with the kids, it seemed that the late evening was the portion of day that I had most freedom to spend a bit of time with him.

His recovery from the shock and trauma of his accident was much slower than that of either Damien or Hedwig and it took a full week of carefully dribbling a diluted meat solution into the crop via a home-made stomach tube. I would have to support his flaccid neck, using gravity to allow the liquid to drain down into his crop in an attempt to prevent him aspirating the material. Then we progressed to crop feeding – carefully forcing tiny balls of minced meat in to his crop and gradually increasing the amount and size. As he slowly became more alert, there never was a time that he seemed intimidated by me and he never showed any sign of aggression although I always stayed immensely respectful of the enormous, elongated talons. My own kids intermittently came to see him, although to them, it wasn't overly unusual to have a strange animal hanging about in the surgery.

In the early days, I tried to minimise contact as much as possible to reduce his stress. At the time, kites were still quite uncommon, and I didn't want a horde of people, however well-intentioned coming to see him so we secretly referred to him as the pigeon! As he got to know me, he slowly regained his feistiness, but when any stranger would enter the room he would slump dramatically on his back in a manner we referred to as his 'dead pigeon act' – an innate survival reflex of his species. I was honoured that he didn't see me as threat and allowed me to see his true cheeky personality!

On one occasion, some months after his arrival, when he had progressed to eating large, roughly cut strips of meat mixed with small feathers to fulfil his dietary requirements and aid his bowel movements, I had him walking loose around the floor of the cattery while I cleaned out his cage. He seemed to enjoy these short outings and he needed to start using his legs and wings, if he was to rehabilitate to any extent.

It was late on a Saturday evening and I had had a call to a Doberman who had pulled a toe nail, deep from the bony area – the pumping blood that ensued brought the owners in to me very quickly, with blood spurting through the home-made bandage all over the back of their car. It was an easy job to sedate 'Moby the Doby' as he was affectionately called. I applied a tourniquet before removing the bandage and cauterising the bleeding vessel. Moby lay slumbering in the recovery kennel as Ciaran made his way from the open door of the cattery into the kennels to investigate. I was in the depths of the cage, scrubbing the incredibly sticky excrement that Ciaran supplied in increasingly voluminous quantities and deposited all over the metal bars when I heard a scuffle and to my horror, turned to see Ciaran, flat on his back, body keeled over in a dramatic death pose. For a split second, I thought that somehow Moby had awoken and escaped and attacked him.

Then I saw the confused-looking Doberman, still safely within the confines of his hospital kennel. He had clearly been disturbed by Ciaran's scuffling and briefly woken from his drug-induced slumber to see a red kite peering in a him and momentarily jumped, startling Ciaran. I often wonder what dogs see when they are sedated or anaesthetised and have visions of them watching pink elephants flying around the room, but poor Moby must have got a fright to see the beak and beady eye of Ciaran and moved suddenly, triggering what I thankfully recognised to be his 'dead pigeon' pose! Within seconds Moby surrendered again to the remnants of the sedative in his blood supply and Ciaran, sensing that the danger was over, picked himself up and hopped off as though nothing untoward had happened.

It was at that stage that I decided he was ready to progress from the confines of the surgery out to a spare wooden stable, which Donal and Jack spent the weekend wiring to be fox-proof and assembling branches to provide a variety of climbing frames and perches.

Difficult as it was for Ciaran to recover physically, his 'mental' rehabilitation was proving even more difficult. It was my mistake that I spent too much time with him, and although I was conscious of not 'taming' him so that in time he could ultimately return to the wild, his need was so intense in the early days that by the time he recovered to any extent he was so comfortable with me that it became difficult to withdraw myself as much as I should have. At around the time that he progressed from eating mince ball to scrag-ends of meat, whenever I would go over to feed him late at night, Ciaran would start to sing as soon as I appeared. It's a song I had never heard before and have never heard since he left, but it was a surprisingly melodic call, definitely similar in certain tones to cries that you will hear when kites fly overheard in the wild, but at the same time very unique and different. I was thrilled the first time he did it and when he didn't do it the next few nights, I thought I had imagined it,. But within a few weeks he would sing every night, initially only when I was on my own, but in time Donal and the kids got to hear it too; I had dragged them over to witness it as I think they thought I was losing it!

I seemed that Ciaran had decided I was his mother, or perhaps his mate – I'm not entirely sure which! While this was terribly flattering to me, at the same time it was not very conducive to getting him back to the wild.

When he first moved from the hospital to the stable I would put him out during the day and take him back in at night for a few weeks to acclimatise him to the change. One evening as I carried him back inside, the surgery phone rang and I reached out with my free hand to answer it. I dealt with the call quickly and reached over to place the phone back on the receiver. Ciaran was perched under my arm as usual and whether I frightened him by the unusual movement or he felt insecure, I don't know, but for whatever reason he struggled and in an instant, gripped my hand and wrist with the talons of his left leg.

They say large-animal practice is dangerous, and in mixed-animal practice I have occasionally been scratched by cats and bitten by dogs, but nothing could compare to the pain of his talons digging deep into my flesh, connecting with the bone in my hand and digging deep into the soft tissue of my wrist on the other side. I was initially stunned, then thought I was going to pass out. It was late in the evening and I was on my own in the surgery, there was no one to help so I had to brace myself and try to prise the razor-sharp talons out of my flesh with one hand while at the same time trying to ensure that his other foot didn't take hold of me. I don't know how long the struggle went on, and at one stage I spotted the large dog nail clippers sitting on the office desk in front of me and was tempted just to cut the talons to free myself from them. But at the time I still hoped that he might some day fly free and if I cut his talons, he would lose his ability to hunt and to perch and do many of the things he needed to do. I have to admit I was tempted, but with a few more attempts, I did finally manage to free myself from his grip and, shaking, carefully place him back in his enclosure.

That episode was a sharp reminder – and one that I needed – that, despite our relationship, Ciaran was, and needed to be, a wild bird. From then, I tried harder to put some distance between us. It was hard when I would go to feed him; I had always hand fed him up to now, as he would simply refuse to eat otherwise. From then on, I would simply place the food on the floor for him and although he was well able to eat, he would sit on his perch and sing forlornly to me as through begging me to feed him. It got to the stage that I would hear his plaintive cry at night in my dreams and see his beady eyes gazing into mine and I was beginning to wonder which of us had the attachment issues! It took almost three weeks, during which time he lost over ten percent of his body weight and I did occasionally give in and hand feed him and he would sing in delight and gaze into my eye as he eagerly took the meat from me, but then I would leave him to it again so by the end of the month he finally surrendered and would fly down and feed for himself.

It had been over six months since his arrival and although I hated to admit it, it was increasingly clear that although

Ciaran was happy and content and thriving, he was not going to be fit for release. Although the bone in his wing had healed, the scarring and adhesions in the muscle tissue meant that he did not have the full, free movement that he needed for perfect hunting flight. It did make me question whether I had done the right thing in putting him through surgery and months of captivity and all that went with it for what should be a free spirit.

The options at that stage were euthanasia or permanent homing in a falconry. Although I questioned what I had done to him, deep down I felt that he was content, even in his confined circumstances, and so he was collected one morning by Marc to travel to his new home.

The red kite reintroduction programme was an incredible success, to the extent that it's hard to drive certain roads of Wicklow without catching a glimpse of one of the magnificent birds. To this day, when I hear the kites calling and circling in the sky, I always think of Ciaran, with mixed feeling of the privilege of having had such an intimate relationship with one of these birds that most people, if they are lucky, get to see in the sky and at the same time of sadness, that whether or not because of my intervention, Ciaran's days of flying free were over.

CHAPTER 18

THE FINAL JOURNEY

I remember sitting in the college canteen one day coming close to our final exams. Our thoughts and conversations were beginning to drift towards life after the five years in the veterinary college. We were discussing the difficulties we might encounter, and one of the girl's biggest concerns was how to deal with the matter of euthanasia.

For sure we knew what injection to give and could describe in some detail the physiological and pharmacological effects of the drug that would ultimately result in the animals' demise but other than that, we had received absolutely no training in how to deal with the client. The longer I am in practice, the more I am convinced that final-year veterinary should include a module on counselling and bereavement with as much emphasis as for clinical and surgical skills. Despite the reassurance on that day in the canteen from one of the lads who boldly declared, 'Sure you're killing them anyway, it's not like it can go wrong', for me euthanasia is probably the most important job we do as vets. In all other cases, if the patient or the owner has a difficult or distressing experience, that day will pass and there will other chances to provide a more pleasant experience, but for the final visit, those last few precious minutes with a beloved pet will often be the most prominent memories for the owner for many years to come.

Many seasoned vets will tell you that 'you get used to it', but I disagree. Veterinary surgeons are near the top of the list of professionals who suffer from alcoholism, drug abuse, divorce and suicide. This, for my money, is as a result of 'getting used to it' – not just the euthanasia, of course, but also the innate hardship of the job, the long hours, the late nights, the demanding clients, the sheer high expectations of an often 'sole practitioner' who is expected to keep up to the standards seen on TV shows where entire teams (and endless finances) support the veterinary hero of the day. When clients ask me if I've watched the latest episode of the current veterinary series, I usually tell them I do it all day so the last thing I want to do when I go home is watch more of it!

Without a doubt, for me, euthanasia, although technically simple, is the most challenging aspect of the job. On some occasions, I've known the pet in question since it was a tiny hairball, though in a way, knowing the pet all its life helps when making the final decision with the owner. Although I always tell owners that they themselves will know when the time has come, still they often look for guidance or at least reassurance that they are doing the right thing. When I come into the story later on in the patient's life, it's harder to know the full story.

Sometimes the answer is black and white – like in the case of an animal hit by a car and in so much pain and beyond any form of repair that although the suddenness of it all is heart-breaking for the owner, there really is no alternative. In other cases it's not so clear cut. Many cats in older age develop kidney failure and many dogs develop lameness or paralysis and these cases can linger uncertainly for months or years.

Often the owner says to me that they hope to come down some morning and find that their beloved pet has passed in their sleep but while I fully understand their sentiment, I have to advise them that it's unlikely to happen. To actually die from these debilitating conditions would require letting the animal regress to such a state of misery that no conscientious owner could bear to watch it without making the phone call. I know, for clients, that picking up the phone to ring is often preceded by hours or even days of self-torture so that when the animal finally passes and is resting peacefully there is almost a sense of relief that it's all over.

As vets, we are simply not trained to support owners through all of this and have to rely on our own personal skills to develop an approach over years of experience that might best help the owner. Many vets who simply don't have those skills, develop the reputation of being heartless or uncaring, even though these are often the vets who suffer the most.

Whenever possible, I try to call to the owners' home once the decision has been made. Allowing the animal to rest in their own bed or beside their own fireplace while the owners sit with them as they gradually drift to sleep, I know, makes it easier for both the pet and the owner. Sometimes, an owner arrives into a busy clinic having made the decision, without telling the nurses and not realising that carrying out a euthanasia in the middle of a clinic is stressful for all involved. Watching a grieving owner carrying out a body to face the lonely drive home is never easy, especially in a waiting room full of exuberant puppies and healthy animals.

One such event springs to mind, from not long after we moved to the new premises. The clinic looked nice and straightforward for the evening. On the appointments screen, I could see a few boosters and routine revisits, plus a new client who had booked in Tabby the cat for a general check-up.

There were still a few more in the waiting room by the time I admitted Tabby. As the elderly lady carried the cat box into the room, I could get the undeniable stench of end-stage kidney failure. Ida told me that her home-help lady who was a client of ours, had recommended that she come as perhaps the cat's teeth needed attention. I could see by how apprehensive my new client was that she already knew there was more going on. She looked so frail that I immediately offered to get her a chair to sit on while I examined the cat. Although she tried to insist she could manage, I went out to the waiting-room to evict

Striper, the practice cat, from her throne and tried to brush the wad of hairs off it, which thankfully matched the chair cover, as I carried it into the consulting room. Ida seemed relieved as she sank into the old chair and didn't speak as I lifted Tabby, unprotestingly, out of the equally ancient cat carrier.

'I found her out in the back garden when she was only a tiny kitten,' Ida told me filling me in on years of history as I examined the emaciated body. 'I don't know what ever happened her mother and I never saw any others, but I took her in and kept her in a cardboard box beside the stove. I had to get a little dropper from the chemist to feed her with, but she was never sick a day in her life. This is the first time I've ever had to bring her to the vet's.'

Without a doubt, it was also going to be her last visit, as I could feel the hardened lumps of kidney clearly jutting out from her bony frame. She objected slightly as I opened her mouth and I almost gagged at the putrid smell. The usual combination of kidney failure and gum disease that go hand-in-hand in so many elderly cats was well beyond any intervention that I could offer.

'When did she eat or drink for you last, Ida?' I asked gently, not wanting to upset the elderly lady who I could picture sitting day after day, offering all sorts of treats to tempt her elderly companion rather than making the visit today which she could clearly see was going to be the end of her sole source of companionship.

'Well, it has been a while,' she admitted. 'I tried a bit of chicken boiled in water, and I got a bit of fresh mince from the butcher, and for a few days she would take a bit of milk if I heated it up, but she has taken nothing for the last few days...' she trailed off silently.

Conscious of the waiting queue outside, but knowing that I couldn't let the little cat go home in such I state, I gently explained her condition to Ida. Her face remained totally expressionless as I explained that Tabby's kidneys had failed and that the only kind option was to let her go to sleep right away.

'I see,' was her only reply. She said no more, and I wasn't sure if she really grasped what I was saying. I continued by explaining that I would give her a tiny injection to sedate her and then when she was fast asleep and unaware of anything, how I would inject and overdose of anaesthetic into her vein.

'I see,' came the reply again.

'Are you okay for me to go ahead with that then, Ida?' I asked gently and she just nodded her consent with her face expressionless.

I offered to place the little cat on her lap as she fell asleep, but she sat without stroking it or talking to it as most owners would do. She clutched the edges of the blanket and remained motionless as I injected the tiny body. Tabby breathed her last and still Ida didn't speak. I took her hand as I removed the lifeless body from her lap and Ida's hands were icy cold.

Wrapping Tabby up carefully in the blanket, I carefully guided Ida out the back door, not wanting to bring her through the busy waiting room. Ida stood looking numbly as I arranged the parcel on her front seat.

'Are you sure you are okay to drive home?' I asked her, thinking to myself that she looked too frail to be driving at the best of times, never mind now.

She nodded and then fumbled to open the driver door. As I handed her her handbag, I took her icy hand once more and then hugged her for a few moments, sensing her total loss and wishing that in some way I could help. She seemed surprised, but held onto me for a few moments before she let go and stiffly got into the car.

With Striper restored to her throne, the rest of the evening was uneventful, with the remaining boosters and a stomach upset. I hoped Ida had made it home safely but didn't feel I could ring to check as apart from the time in the clinic I had never met her before.

It was about a week later that a card arrived in the post. The carefully stepped in address and the spidery handwriting instantly identified it as being from an elderly person.

It took a few minutes to decipher the shaky hand as Ida wrote to thank me for helping her to make the decision to let Tabby go to sleep. She apologised if she had let her go too far, but explained that she was her only companion. I was stunned as I read the closing lines.

'Thank you for the kindness of your hug as I left. It is the only time I remember being hugged in my life and I will always treasure it,' she ended.

※ ※ ※

Thankfully, not all euthanasias are so poignant.

It was only a few months after that another elderly client arrived in, but this one with his wife and two adult sons. I had known their two collies since first opening the practice, so although I had missed their early years, I felt I knew them well enough to be part of the decision when the time came. The two dogs, Sally and Sheba, had enjoyed a great life, ranging freely over the owners' vast estate by day and slumbering in front of a stove in the kitchen by night. Strangely, they had never so much as looked at sheep and so had enjoyed great freedom over the years.

Slowly, with the passing of time, age had caught up with the two buddies so instead of galloping around the field, they were more likely to go for an occasional potter before returning to the comforts of the kitchen.

The start of the end came one evening when Mr Lambert, as he always referred to himself, rang to say Sheba had collapsed and was unable to get up.

'I suppose that's the end of the road for her so,' he stated matter-of-factly.

But it wasn't. Although Sheba was the younger of the two by at least three years, it seemed she had suffered a minor stroke,

221

but responded well to a few days' hospitalisation and returned home to Sally on long-term, but low-dose, medication. Her check-ups became more frequent, with the minor issues that can be expected with advancing years, but still she enjoyed her life roasting herself in front the fire and shuffling around the front garden with her buddy for a long time after. But the day came when despite increasing her medication, Sheba was no longer able to get up. I always tell clients that if a dog is sleeping comfortably, eating and drinking and able to get up and shuffle out to the toilet then, in dog terms, they are still enjoying life. Sheba was no longer able to get up and refused food for the first time since her hospitalisation.

As I drove up the long, stony driveway, I wasn't expecting any high emotion or drama as the Lamberts, although taking excellent care of their dogs, were usually quite matter-of-fact about life in general. Sheba looked tired, stretched at the stove and I was glad to be able to help her as I injected the sedation which would allow me to give the intravenous anaesthetic without any distress to her. Sally sat nearby, but was not overly interested in the entire proceeding. Although there was no great show of emotion, I sensed a bit of friction between Mr Lambert and his wife, Emily, and the two adult sons but I didn't comment

'Poor old Sally,' I said as I injected Sheba. 'She'll miss her buddy.'

'Well, we have decided,' spoke out Mr Lambert, 'to get the two dogs put to sleep together. Kindest thing to do,' he affirmed.

I must have looked as stunned as I felt as Mr Lambert immediately interjected, 'It's been discussed and decided,' and immediately I understood the tension that had been simmering since my arrival. Clearly Emily and the sons didn't agree, but Mr Lambert was always in charge of everything in his kingdom. In hindsight, I recalled that all decision had to be 'run by Dad', in the same way that all the cheques were signed by himself only.

Thankfully, however, I was not in a position where I had to succumb to Mr Lambert's wishes and I knew before I spoke that it was going to be a case of four against one not even counting Sally whose fate was being decided in front of her.

'I'm sorry, Mr Lambert. I really don't think that's a good idea. Sally is still in good health, even though she is older than Sheba. Of course she will miss her, but I know from experience that in time, with plenty of attention and maybe looking at getting another dog she will go on to live out her natural life span.'

There was total silence as Mr Lambert took in what I was saying and I noticed tears welling up in Emily's eyes. The sons shuffled awkwardly against the kitchen countertop, clearly avoiding Mr Lambert's eyes.

I could see that he was not pleased with my interference, but before he had a chance to speak, I continued.

'As a vet, I can only ever justify euthanasia if the animal is suffering and that's certainly not the case with Sally.' As far as

I was concerned the discussion was over.

Sally, on hearing her name, thumped her tail on the tiled floor as though agreeing.

'Bloody ridiculous if you ask me,' he muttered and there was tension for a few minutes as nobody spoke. By then however, Sheba was feeling the effects of the sedation so I carried on with the job and all the attention was back on Sheba as I clipped her vein and she took a few slow breaths as I injected the blue liquid into her vein.

Sally ignored the entire proceedings, but as I checked Sheba's heart for the last time, I turned to Emily and said, 'If I was you I would leave Sheba here with Sally for a few hours before you bury her. Dogs can understand, in a way that we don't, what is going on.'

Mr Lambert ignored the conversation as he busied himself writing out the cheque, the cost of which had already been carefully negotiated some weeks previously. The eldest of the two sons sat down and hugged the remains of Sheba and I could just about make him out as he muttered, 'We'll stick him in the grave with you if he's not careful!'

I didn't see them until a few months later when they made an appointment to vaccinate a young terrier that had apparently been found straying nearby. Sally, although looking aged beside her new, young companion, looked delighted with herself as she busied herself keeping an eye on the slightly more troublesome terrier. Emily was beaming and as they left the consulting room. As Mr Lambert handed me the carefully signed cheque for the consultation fee, he coughed a few times to clear his throat before gruffly throwing out the few words, 'I suppose you were right.'

'I'm delighted, Mr Lambert. Really I am,' I assured him as we shook hands.

※ ※ ※

Some animals, however, have less dignified endings.

Although I tried to engage myself as little as possible in anything other than small animals, on occasions I was called to deal with something outside my area of supposed expertise. One of my clients reared poultry as a sideline and his latest batch of forty chickens had started to dwindle at an alarming rate. His description of their symptoms didn't ring any bells as they would dramatically lose weight and then drop dead over a three- to four-day period. I spoke to a colleague who was far more knowledgeable than I on such matters and she suggested carrying out a post-mortem on a couple of the birds as they died to see if that would shed any light on the matter. John agreed to bring in the next casualty and only the next day I saw his jeep pulling up with, I assumed, the latest victim. As it was a hot day, he opened the back of the jeep and sat resting on the opened door while chatting to a few of the clients. I could see the poultry box in amongst the sacks of hen feed and whatever else. As the nurses were busy down the back washing a particular obstreperous terrier, I went out to take the luckless bird from John, to save him waiting.

'I'll be back to you in one minute,' I assured Eileen who sat with her spaniel, waiting for his ears to be cleaned.

'Oh, take your time. I'm in no rush at all,' she replied. I could see that she thought that I was skipping the queue due to some sense of urgency with the patient in the poultry box.

As I passed back through the waiting room she tried to catch a glimpse of the patient and could clearly see some feathers sticking out.

'I'll let you know as soon as we have any news,' I called back to John over my shoulder.

'I do hope your chicken gets better soon,' Eileen added encouragingly, as myself and John made eyes at each other, silently agreeing not to enlighten her any further.

⁂

These small moments of lightness are essential in a job where you never know what you are going to encounter from one moment to the next.

CHAPTER 19

VERMIN!

Although the vast majority of our patients at Clover Hill were small animals, and even the cats getting a very poor look-in compared to the dogs, occasionally there was a chance to work with some more unusual characters. Edward, my long-eared donkey buddy who I got to meet on a relatively regular basis, lived with a Highland bullock, a few horses, two goats, a variety of birds and Biddy the fox.

Biddy had been hand-reared when her mother had been killed on the road. As the only surviving cub, she became very accustomed to her new life and although shy with strangers, settled in well to enjoy life in her little commune. When the occasional duck or hen started to disappear during daylight, her free ranging had to be confined somewhat and at night she was safely confined in her own personal den, as much for her own safety as that of the birds. Although the dogs regarded her with suspicion, she enjoyed the same food as them, although in respect to her wild origins, her Sunday night treat was usually the remains of the ray wings from the local chipper which she always relished.

My only previous significant encounter with a fox was back in the early days of my time in mixed practice, long before the arrival of the kids.

I was behind the office desk, wading my way through signing what seemed like an endless batch of TB cards, when one of the local beef farmers arrived in. Unlike many of the clients, Declan was one of those farmers who appeared to have little interest in his stock apart from their economic potential. Visits to the yard were always frustrating, and I usually left feeling like I hadn't done my job well.

On this occasion, Declan was rushing, and I was grateful at least not to have to engage in a lengthy discussion in relation to his latest bill.

Without as much as a glance at me, he dumped a tattered feed sack, tied with a length of baling twine, on the countertop.

'I found this vermin on the side of the road,' he said, already making his way back out the road. 'Would have put a bullet in it myself, but I'm on the way to the mart with cattle and I don't want it stinking in the truck all day.'

I didn't even manage to respond as he was already on his way back out the front door. 'And don't be putting any charge on the bill for that one,' he threw in as the heavy front door swung shut behind him.

'It takes all sorts to make the world, doesn't it?' I heard from the side-counter. I looked up to see Jack Doyle, one of our more popular farmer clients, waiting patiently for a prescription. I had been so engrossed in my TB certs that I hadn't even noticed him come in. Jack ran a serious dairy operation, but in contrast to Declan, he personally knew each cow and their offspring, and he and his two stock-men minded them better then he looked after himself. With Jack, nothing was ever too much trouble, and he always listened intently to any advice I could offer, although I was quite sure that with his years of experience and his obvious passion for the job, any advice I could give him would be of little value.

'So what d'ye think is in the sack?' he enquired inquisitively as it mysteriously began to make its way across the countertop.

'I've no idea,' I replied honestly.

Placing my hands on the old-style bag, I could at least feel a warm furry body, roughly the size of a small dog, but it was the smell that alerted me that something was different. Cautiously untying the twine and peering in, I was enthralled to find the bright eyes of a young fox staring back at me. Suddenly realising that I was in the wide open space of the front office, I withdrew to the small enclosed consulting room with Jack following closely on my heels, reluctant to miss anything of interest. Turning off the bright surgery light so that only the dim bulb remained, I carefully took hold of the quivering animal by the scruff of its neck and withdrew it from its haven. Jack feigned horror when he saw my patient.

'There won't be a chicken safe in Wicklow. Vermin for sure!' he retorted, but I could see by his twinkling eyes that he too was fascinated. The young, but almost fully-grown little vixen, allowed me to gently examine her. Although she was clearly shocked, the only significant injury I could find was a fractured jaw but only the little joint, joining the right and left lower jaw bones. I knew from my orthopaedic training that it would be a matter of minutes under anaesthetic to place a piece of wire, using the lower canine teeth to prevent it from slipping in the few weeks that it would take to heal in such a young and otherwise healthy animal.

'Ah, now don't tell me you're even thinking of trying to fix it up,' said Jack throwing his eyes up to heaven and at the same time reaching out to stroke the sleek head. Two bright eyes honed in on us, as I muttered something non-committal, quickly wrapping her up in the bag again as I heard Seamus, the boss, coming in the front door.

My plan was foiled, as Jack a longterm, fellow IFA member, and friend of Seamus, opened the door to beckon him in.

'I hope you don't have any serious cattle calls lined up, Seamus. Nurse Nightingale here has an important surgery to do, so you'll be on your own!'

Seamus clearly wasn't in such good humour. He took one look in the bag and said, 'Make sure it's gone out of here by this evening.'

I took that as an open invitation to abandon signing the

TB cards. Once the little fox was peacefully sleeping, inhaling the mixture of anaesthetic gas and oxygen, it did only take minutes to wire the jaw. Vermin, as I affectionately called her in respect to the good Samaritan who brought her in, came home with me in the back of the car that evening. Over the few weeks that Vermin stayed with us, in one of the stables that were vacant for the summer, I watched with fascination how, although reasonably docile to handle, she retained that fiery look in her eye of a truly wild animal.

The surgery to remove the wire was even quicker than it had been to insert and less than a month after her arrival, Vermin made the return journey to the outskirts of the practice and I took a detour on the way down to release her close to Declan's farm. When I opened the box, she stepped out delicately, taking a few sniffs of the hopefully familiar environment, whiskers twitching dramatically and then she turned and looked at me and I got a last glimpse of the those innately wild eyes before she darted off into the hedgerow and with a last rustling of the bushes, she was gone.

It was a few years later that I got to know Biddy the fox. It was always the very specific smell of her that would bring me back to Vermin and I often wondered how she or her potential offspring were doing in the wild. I never had much cause to see

Biddy as she was remarkably healthy, but I would often drop in to say hello to her, particularly if the kids were with me as they were always fascinated to see a real live fox, far from the demonised villains of their bedtime stories.

Although she always carried the odour peculiar to her kind, on one occasion as I peered into her night time pen, the smell was clearly more pungent and Karen was concerned that apart from the smell, she was having to refill the water bowl on an increasingly frequent basis.

It's not easy to get a urine sample from a fox, but Karen was adept and knew her animals well so within a day or two the required sample arrived and my suspicion was confirmed that Biddy had a raging urinary-tract infection. Although nothing was licenced for urinary tract infections in foxes, I was reasonable confident that a similar combination that was used successfully for dogs would suffice and sure enough, within two weeks, although Biddy refused to produce another sample, the smell was back to normal and the water bowl was lasting the full day.

My secret pleasure at my fox cure was short lived as within two weeks the symptoms were back. As we had been unable to get a sample giving the all clear, I assumed that the course had been insufficient and so repeated it for a longer duration. This time, Karen was determined to get a sample and even after a longer course, although much improved, the sample was still showed some blood and white cells. A microscopic examination confirmed the result. I knew now that, at this stage although again Biddy seemed much improved, she would need an ultrasound examination of her kidneys, bladder and uterus. Usually animals would come to the clinic for ultrasound examination for both convenience and more important to protect the hideously expensive piece of machinery that I could in no way economically justify having in a small, one vet practice. For Biddy, I made an exception, although not without some concern, watching the machine perched on top of a barrel outside her pen for the duration of the examination. Biddy was remarkable co-operative as I clipped and cleaned her abdomen. When the cold gel was applied, Biddy started to pant as Karen, down on her knees, held her securely.

'I've absolutely no idea what you're looking at!' Karen proclaimed as the black and white images appeared on the screen.

'Either have I!' I laughed, freely admitting this this was my first and probably last ultrasound examination of a fox. Thankfully the three large white spherical shaped surrounded by the black shadow of the urine in the bladder made it blatantly evident the cause of Biddy's recurrent infection was the bladder stones. I was less enthusiastic as I realised that due to their size, surgery was going to the only option.

Whatever about an ultrasound examination, in my inexperienced hands, anaesthesia and surgery was a little more daunting! Although I had anaesthetised Vermin some years previously, it was a very short procedure and as her ultimate destination at the time had been euthanasia, it was worth the risk.

I explained my concerns to Karen. While her confidence was flattering, it in ways made it worse. Her own father, Bill Bennet, had been a vet who tragically had passed away at a young age. From everything I had heard about him from older colleagues, it seemed that the man had a natural gift that went way beyond his academic learning, along with a compassion that made him a favourite with both patients and clients.

The surgery was booked for a Sunday, as it was likely that Biddy would have the place to herself. She walked in on a lead with Karen, looking almost as apprehensive as I felt. After Karen had left, I sat with her in a darkened room, waiting for the sedative to take effect – noting how her heart rate slowed as the medication slowly took effect, almost mirroring the increase in my own!

'Come on now, Bill, give us a hand here,' I muttered under my breath, imploring the help of my long-departed colleague as I drew up a carefully measured dose of anaesthetic. The anaesthetic induction which I had devised after consultation with other vets and what was termed as 'anecdotal evidence' from the drug companies was remarkably smooth so before long, with Biddy intubated, I was engrossed in the surprisingly standard-looking abdomen, surgically prepped under the green operating drapes. As I focused on packing around the bladder with sterile surgical swabs before incising into the thickened and inflamed looking wall, making an incision big enough to remove the stones, I almost forgot about the unusual odour, and the giveaway bushy tail hanging down from under the heated surgical bed. The three stones were easy to locate and by the time I was placing the final skin incisions, while Biddy's heart rate and respiration rate remained stable, mine had almost returned to normal.

Having administered appropriate pain relief and cut off the gaseous anaesthetic supply leaving Biddy inhaling a supply of pure oxygen, within minutes, she was sitting up, eye-balling me and apparently totally unfazed by her experience. As kidney and bladder stones can often be prevented by dietary change, she was discharged later that evening on a commercial prescription diet, but as she had made it to almost eight years of age by the time of her surgery, we did agree to make a concession so that evening she was tucked up, back in her usual den with her Sunday night treat of ray wings from the local chipper!

CHAPTER 20

CLIENTS VS THE PATIENTS

I f you had asked me at the tender age of six why I wanted to become a vet, I would have told you that it was because I loved animals. I might not have admitted that it was also because I didn't have a lot of time for people. It was many years before I realised that the animals came with owners attached. As a child, my main companions' were a black spaniel called Crackers and a black horse called Setanta. Unfortunately, both were imaginary. As a teenager, I underwent the usual ritual of three weeks in the Gaeltacht and came back with photos of a stray dog that used to hang around the school campus, seals swimming at the local beach and flocks of sheep.

I definitely had a better ability to communicate with animals than people. I even met Donal through spending most of my teenage afternoons in a field that his father rented to keep their ponies in. It really was the ponies I was interested in!

Animals always inspired me in a way that people couldn't.

They seemed to have a depth to them that, to me, most people lacked. To this day, as a client tells me their version of what is going on with the patients, while I do listen, I pay more heed to what the animal is telling me. I find that although their form of communication is more subtle, it is always more accurate.

As a child I was shy, but could talk endlessly with or about animals. When in college we came to our clinical years, when we had to actually carry out clinical consultations, I was apprehensive at first, but quickly found that, for the duration of that consultation, as the client's only interest was in the animal, communication became easy. It was as though the animals themselves acted as silent mediators between myself and the client and so quickly I found myself able to develop a rapport with the human owners.

In our final year, we were assigned patients that we had to care for for the duration of their stay at the hospital. When the cases were being handed out one day, a particular large, elderly unneutered male German Shepherd was on the list. I had met the dog during his initial assessment and, although he was terribly nervous and clearly way beyond his comfort zone, there was nothing about his temperament that concerned me. I gladly volunteered to take him when he was admitted for prostate surgery.

Knowing him to be anxious, I came to college early for the week, so that I could have some time to just sit with him and gain his trust before the daily madness started. Shep trusted me. That in itself was more than ample reward for my extra care, but the icing on the cake came when I was summoned from the canteen one afternoon by no less than the head professor of the surgical department. Although on paper I was a model student, myself and himself didn't always see eye-to-eye and had a few strained run-ins during the course of the clinical year. I couldn't think exactly why I might have been summoned but was sure it wasn't a good thing.

As it happened, the professor was on his daily ward rounds and, as Shep was due to be discharged that afternoon, he was anxious to check him over before signing off the discharge papers. But Shep was having none of it. While the students might have had to bite their tongues and succumb to the wishes of the professor, usually issued in abrupt measure, Shep had no need to pass his finals and was more inclined to bite the professor.

When I arrived at the kennels, the professor was irately pacing up and down the kennels while Shep, by now totally fraught, was lunging at the kennel bars, feeling totally threatened by the animosity. One of the nurses who had seen the time I had spent with Shep had suggested calling me, and there was nothing the professor could do about it. I hope I was able to supress my glee as I quietly asked the professor to wait outside to give me a minute to calm the patient. I closed the door behind him and sat down at the kennel in front of Shep who within minutes was lying quietly enough for me to open the door. I sat to the side of the kennel until he came and lay his head on my lap and didn't rush myself as I chatted to him for a while before slipping the lead over his head and walking him calmly to where the professor was waiting. Shep shook, but allowed himself to be examined as I continued to speak in gentle, soothing tones that I knew was driving my future examiner crazy!

When it came to doing our final-year presentations, I couldn't resist picking Shep as my case study, glad that he had made a complete recovery.

Probably the biggest disappointment with a career in veterinary medicine is that once you are immersed in the frantic pace of life, there is no longer that time to spend getting to know and gain the trust of the patient. The hours I had spent as a student and before were simply no longer available. On many occasions, when a nervous patient arrives in a busy clinic, there is no option but to carry on without taking the time to get to know them. In some cases, with time that trust comes in a way that fascinated me. Surprisingly, it is often after an animal is admitted for an overnight stay that they get over their fear of coming to the vets. In the early days of Clover Hill, Smokey, a young Glen of Imaal terrier spent a few nights with us with gastric issues, which had required relatively major surgery. He clearly enjoyed his stay so enormously that for many years after, on arrival for any routine visit, he would abandon his owner and run down towards the kennels as though checking in for another stay.

Despite their anxiety coming in, in general the animals are way easier to deal with than the owners. On one occasion, as I examined the eyes of an elderly Bearded Collie, the owners were distraught when I told them that Oscar was almost blind. Oscar, of course, had acclimatised to his condition so well that the owners had not noticed but even though I explained this to them, they were inconsolable to the extent that the unfortunate Oscar who, five minutes previously, had been perfectly happy, started to become anxious, clearly wondering what tragedy had overcome his beloved owners that had upset them so much. So often, I find myself recommending that the owners observe the dog's behaviour so that when a lump turns out to be potentially cancerous, I encourage them to be like their dog – perfectly happy, with no anticipation of what may or indeed may not ever happen.

Amputation is thankfully a rare salvage procedure that we recommend only when a limb can't be saved and although radical in some sense, it is usually well tolerated by the animal. The main difficulty with this seemingly barbaric surgery is in convincing the owners that it is the best option. I can fully understand the owners' apprehension as, even to me, it seems such an extreme option and every three-legged cat or dog running around Wicklow haunts me a personal failure. But this is only my issue and really nothing to do with the quality of life of the pets.

It's always a delicate balance discussing the surgery with owners as I always try to simply present the options and allow an owner to make an informed choice as to what is best for their pet. Not uncommonly, when presenting the option of amputation the initial reaction from the owner is to request putting the animal to sleep. It takes much talk and reassurance to convince the owners that such drastic measures are in general not warranted.

Kids always strike me as being more like animals than their parents and it is usually the younger generation who are more open to suggestion that the world-weary adults. Tiddles, an eighteen-month-old neutered cat arrived in late one night after being found by a neighbour. Whatever led her to an encounter with a car, she had clearly come out second best. Despite the dragging hind limb, Tiddles was still feeling feisty and had miraculously avoided any other injuries. After lengthy discussion with the three primary-school boys – Rory, Fiachra and Lorcan – who owned her and their mother, Marie, the next day I attempted to place an intramedullary pin to repair the fractured femur. Unfortunately, although on the radiographs it looked as though this might be a reasonable option, as soon as I attempted to place the pin in the proximal fragment, the length of bone simply crumbled into fragments. Although this is a rare occurrence, it reminded me of a similar situation some years previously, when I had attempted to pin the wing of a very elderly gander who had a significant career as a film star. The bone had simply splintered into fragments and the unfortunate gander had to be euthanised. It took many weeks before tiny white feathers stopped appearing in random places in the theatre.

Thankfully, in Tiddles case, due to her young age and agility, amputation was going to be a suitable option. The only difficulty was in convincing the mother, who was understandably shocked at the sudden and drastic change of plan. Her main concern was how the three boys would take it. From previous experience, I knew that once Tiddles was back home and able to demonstrate to the kids that life was good, the lads in question would have no difficulty in adapting to a three-limbed pet.

When the very happy three-limbed Tiddles was ready to go home a couple of days later, the lads were clearly enthralled by the remains of the shaved limb, and their main question was in relation to the fate of the missing fourth limb.

As vets, we are in the enviable position of regularly receiving thank-you cards and gifts from grateful owners. Sometimes I wonder how we are so much appreciated when other professions work just as hard with no obvious thanks. Probably the best thank-you cards we receive come from children, and over the years I have a collection of the more special ones that sometimes just remind me why we do what we do. On this occasion, when Tiddles returned for a wound check, her minders brought a card. The laminated card was clearly the work of her real owners and bore a picture of myself (I assume) coloured in in full surgical green with a very impressive green surgical cap. In my hand was a large corrugated saw, dripping with blood, while Tiddles was pictured lying dramatically on the surgical table, looking on, watching the entire proceedings. On the floor beside me was drawn a rectangular box, clearly labelled as the 'limb bin'.

Clearly the kids had got over the trauma of the surgery and Tiddles herself was well on the way back to three-legged normality. We kept the card in the surgery for a long time, despite questioning looks from some of the more sensitive clients!

So definitely, the patients were usually the easiest to deal with, followed by the kids and lastly the adults.

In the same way as I learned to observe what animals were telling me with their silent language, I definitely think they also taught me how to deal with people. Some animals have better people-management skills than others and I found over the years that older animals seemed to have it all worked out. Treating older animals can at times be more rewarding than treating younger animals, as they seem to have developed a sensitivity and intuition that younger animals are simply too busy for. To me, animals age with way more grace and dignity than many people I know, although there are of course exceptions.

I was lucky that especially when I have treated a particular pet over a long period of time, owners trust that we have their best interests at heart. If a young dog suffers a severe injury, it is reasonable to me to perform invasive and potentially stressful procedures, knowing that there is good potential that the dog will have many years to benefit from the intervention. When an old dog is clearly struggling and then develops another major injury or illness, although I outline all the available options, I normally advise owners that it is in the best interests of the pet to keep them happy as long as possible, rather than alive as long as possible. Sometimes starting into major surgical intervention or medications that require lots of monitoring and follow with a long list of potential side effects is really just a human reaction wanting to hold on to the pet for as long as possible regardless of the quality of life for the pet. Each individual case is different and each pet has to be assessed for their own unique requirements, but in general the animals themselves are way more accepting of ageing and dying than the owners.

Working with older pets becomes a three-way bond between owner, pet and vet that lasts until the final breath is released. It is in these situation that I realise what I have learned from my patients in teaching owners to trust my good intention. Although of course in some ways it is understandably a matter of avoiding being the one to make a decision, it amazes me how often an owner will ask, 'What would you do if it was your pet.' In ways, it's a silly question and I can't be honest and tell them if it was my own beloved pet facing terminal illness that of course I would fall apart and hope that someone else would guide me! Although I always try to allow the owner to come to the decision for themselves, in some cases, particularly if the pet deteriorates quickly and is suffering, I often find that by telling them if it was my pet I would let them go, they will allow the decision to be made.

Over the years in practice, I have found it very humbling to realise just how much trust an owner will place in our hands. As a new graduate it was totally intimidating but at least I knew that I didn't know enough to deserve their confidence. As time went on, I gradually became more confident in not only outlining the options, but also in guiding the owner as to what would be the best option for them and their pet.

Probably the best skill I learned was to know what I didn't know and to have the confidence to tell owners that I didn't know. All new graduates feel under pressure to prove them-selves and I always tried to have an answer for everything, but as real-life experience padded the scant knowledge I had learnt from the text books, I became much more comfortable acknowledging when something was beyond my skill. At that stage, I would more than happily do some research or get in touch with someone more senior than myself for advice or, in some cases, refer the patient to specialist or referral hospital. What fascinated me was how often, having explained the reason for referral, the owner would still want me to continue looking after the medical case or to perform a surgery that I was simply not well enough equipped for or experience at.

In the early days, I probably put myself under a lot of pressure, trying to look after more cases and patients than I was able for, feeling somewhat obliged to meet people's expectations of me. Again, with increasing experience I learnt to gently refuse to do something myself that I knew someone else could do better apart from cases where the cost of referral was prohibitive to the extent that the animal would be left untreated.

※ ※ ※

In all walks of life, things go wrong. Misdiagnosis, adverse drug reaction, simple human error, all for a variety of reasons are an unfortunate reality of life. Somebody's beloved pet has to be the one that is listed as being a 0.01 percent risk of a particular reaction. More often than not there is no logical explanations for these outcomes. When things do go wrong I am usually more gutted than the owner and can fully understand how upset or angry they would be.

On one such occasion, we had a relatively calm and quiet day at the surgery. The clinic was nicely paced with plenty of time to chat to owners and patients which was always nice, especially with new clients.

With only two patients for surgery, we stopped for a cup of tea which was always a welcome interlude in the day. Although the Labrador for spaying was already overweight at nine months, the surgery was very routine. Apart from her, the only other surgical patient was Squire, a spaniel who had developed a cyst on his lower eyelid that although relatively benign-looking, was causing him considerable irritation. As it was getting bigger, the owner was happy to take my advice that surgical removal would be the best option.

I almost opted for simple sedation and removal under local anaesthetic, but with Squire sedated, I was better able to examine the lesion and although in the consulting room it had looked relatively superficial, it was actually invading well into the tissue of the eyelid so I decided I would carry out the procedure under full anaesthetic enabling me to remove a small wedge of the eyelid to ensure that the entire mass would be removed with little change of regrowth. I had already discussed both of these option with Peter, the owner, on the day I had examined Squire and he had signed consent for either procedure so there was no need to make further contact as he was happy to let me decide which was best.

With Squire sleeping peacefully on the theatre table,

taking slow steady breaths of the mix of oxygen and anaesthetic gas through his endotracheal tube, I filled his eye with a lubricating gel to protect it as I carefully clipped around the eye and disinfected the area. Preparing for eye surgery is always tricky, but before long I was happily dissecting out the cyst. I always enjoyed suturing the edges of the eyelid as it has to be exact to ensure that once the hair grown back there is no obviously abnormality especially as the dogs eyes are such an expressive feature of their face. Once I was happy that the margin of the eyelid was exactly apposed, I quickly sutured the outer and inner eyelid and carefully flushed the eye with gently heated saline to remove any blood. Squire was soon back in the recovery kennels while I went to fill in his surgery report and discharge sheet before going for lunch.

With my back turned to Squire, I was startled when I heard a loud bang. I turned around to see him having a full-blown epileptic seizure. In the early days, when anaesthetic agents were not what they are now, animals could have small seizures while going to sleep or waking up, but modern anaesthetic agents just don't result in these reactions, and this was a major seizure, so aggressive, that I had to quickly restrain Squire, putting most of my weight across his body to stop him from damaging himself within the confines of the kennel.

Although such a dramatic reaction is an incredibly rare occurrence, the theatre is always prepared for these emergency situations. Within seconds, Amanda was handing me the emergency crash box from which I drew up a dose of anti–seizure medications. She had to use considerable effort to hold him steady as I injected it into his intravenous cannula. Soon he was relaxed and breathing normally again, but his heart rate was high and his mucous membrane colour was poor.

The prospect of lunch was now history as we wheeled the anaesthetic machine into the kennels enabling us to oxygenate Squire to help his recovery.

Despite the sedative, in less than five minutes Squire was seizuring again. It took a higher dose this time to control the seizure, so once he was calm I connected a giving set so that we could allow continuous medication to be administered with more ease. Usually an adverse reactions after an anaesthetic resolves quickly but it was well over an hour later with Squire still needing continuous medications that I was able to leave him with Amanda and ring Peter. He answered with his usual bright and cheery voice but quickly became silent as I explained how despite the routine surgery, Squire was in difficulty now. There was a silence as I came to end, not knowing what more I could tell him other than we were doing everything we could to stabilise him. After a few seconds, Peter asked in quiet, unfamiliar tones, 'So tell me, is he going to pull through or not?'

'I don't honestly know, Peter,' I answered. 'I've never seen such a severe reaction and we are having difficulty stabilising him. He just doesn't seem to be responding as I would expect.'

Again there was a pause, before Peter spoke again.

'Just do whatever you have to do either way. I'll leave all the decisions in your hands. If you think he's not going to make it just put him to sleep.'

This time it was me that paused, not knowing what to say, but before I could think of anything, Peter had hung up. I couldn't blame him, as the healthy dog that he had left in for routine surgery that morning was now critical.

Squire did pull though, although it was well after tea-time before we could leave him and I wearily made my way over to the house for a quick sandwich before I headed back to the evening clinic. I kept him in overnight to monitor him, but he never looked back. Peter was delighted when he came to collect him the next morning.

'You're causing me a lot of drama for no reason,' he told Squire, clearly relieved to see him in one piece. 'I was thinking to myself after you rang yesterday to say it wasn't looking good for him. If it was anyone else, I would have been raging, but at least I knew when he was with you, whatever happened he would be in the best hands.'

I didn't know whether to cry or to hug him, but was just more relieved than anything to see Squire going home in one piece.

As they were going out the door, I called after them.

'Just one thing, Peter. If that cyst grows back again, it's staying there!'

One vet I knew had come up with a novel scheme to motivate staff, so that instead of offering a Christmas bonus, he allowed them to choose ten clients they would throw out of the practice. Over lunch one day, many months after Squire's episode, we sat down and tried to imagine who we would pick. Despite a client register that by now was well over three thousand, between us we couldn't think of ten people to choose. After the first five, we were sort of stuck, as most suggestions after that had some sort of redeeming quality that gave them a free pass. We actually spent much more time then discussing how many lovely clients we had.

Despite the drama and the ups and downs, and despite the fact that as a child, I only wanted to work with animals and have nothing to do with people, the years spent dealing with the owners had made me over time grow to like people a whole lot more.

EPILOGUE

It seemed like very recently that I had first stood on the steps of the University College Dublin Veterinary Hospital campus. I can still clearly remember that first morning of college, having first gone up the wrong road in a vain attempt to find the place, then finally finding my way to the large metal gates and taking a deep breath as I walked through the entrance.

I can remember the feeling of almost awe and reverence, that I had finally made it through those gates, after the setback of illness and three attempts at the Leaving Certificate before I finally got that much-coveted offer in the post for VET MED DN005. The weeks leading up to college had seemed surreal, and finally I was here. Professor Mc Geady, the dean at the time, terrified us all with a welcoming talk on how tough the course was going to be. If we weren't one hundred per cent committed to it, then to walk away now without wasting any further time. I was going nowhere. I was sure that this was the path for me.

Despite the fact that in our first year, we spent half the week in the general campus in Belfield, only making it to the Balls-bridge veterinary college mid-week, we soon slotted in. Being such a small faculty, there was perhaps a closer bond between us, especially as the years went by and we were divided into increasingly smaller groups for more advanced clinical work. My clinical group in final year consisted of only five of us – four from Cork and me from Dublin, but now living in Wicklow. By the end of final year, I had developed as a good a Cork accent as any of them and still, some twenty years later, find myself lapsing into the Cork lilt in times of extreme duress!

I remember the vet ball in first year, only a few months into our time in the college. When myself and Donal made to leave in the early hours of the morning, not partaking of the college bus, one of the final year lads stopped him in the corridor while another took me carefully aside to ask was I sure I was okay going off on my own with him!

Far more difficult than the time in college, were the first few months in practice, when the stark reality of the road ahead became clear in a way that no text books or college lectures could have prepared us. It was surprisingly lonely to suddenly be in charge. Having gone from seeing practice in a vibrant family business for much of my time in college or from sitting in tutorials with a group of students you had worked with for years, to suddenly being out on the road or in a clinic or makeshift surgery was tougher than any college exams.

The expectations of clients were high. A vet was a vet. Many didn't seem to see or care that you did not have the twenty years' experience of the guy you worked for. And in fairness, they were paying the same money for the job, so they were right to have high expectations. The animals, be they farm animals or beloved pets, had the right to good treatment. No one wanted them to bear the brunt of our inexperience. And even more so, I, and I am sure most of my colleagues, had even higher expectations.

Since the tender age of six, I had decided to be the best vet I could possibly be. When I first qualified, I didn't see that even years of study and of seeing practice could not give me the skills that only time and practice would bring. To this day, the most depressing day of my life was the day I qualified as a vet. The hard work and the stress and anticipation and the excitement of all the years had all bundled into the morning when I took the bus up the N11 for one of the last times the get my results. I was reasonably confident that I had got through, but somehow I felt that deep down, having the piece of paper in my hands would in some way magically transform the little I had learnt into a state of all-knowingness.

Seeing my name on the board was, of course, a relief – but then it hit me that that was all it was. There wasn't going to be a magical moment of transformation. All I had was what I had learned and my fumbling practice, and a huge awareness of all the gaps in my now supposed 'professional expertise'.

I didn't even go out to celebrate that night as I fell into the depths of despair over what suddenly to me seemed like a total failure. And over the next month, while we waited to graduate, suddenly for the first time in my life I felt like I had no focus. In that month, instead of looking forward to starting work, I become more and more anxious and apprehensive about the whole thing. And of course when I did start, it wasn't all smooth sailing. Things went wrong. I screwed up. Animals didn't do the things that it said they did in the text book. Surgeries didn't look like they did in the pictures. I quickly discovered that the most difficult and unpredictable animal was the two-legged one! To this day I maintain that final year veterinary should include modules on people care as much as animal care.

But slowly, with time and with experience, things started to settle. 'Routine treatment' began to actually *feel* routine. I became more optimistic in my prognosis. I subdued the urge to whisper in surgery.

Bitch spays are probably the biggest fear of small-animal vets after graduation. Although now, with increasing specialisation and multi-vet practices, it is less common, when I first qualified, it was not uncommon for the first bitch spay a new graduate would carry out to be in a clinic and unsupervised; I myself had undergone this ordeal in my student days. Although it is a routine surgery, it can still be tricky – especially if the dog is large or overweight. The biggest risk is of haemorrhage either during or after the surgery. For years the first thing I, and I suspect many of my colleagues, would do would be to check if there were any spays booked in for the day. A phone call in the evening from an owner to say the patient was bleeding would send me into a panic.

I don't know how long it was after I qualified, but I clearly remember the night that I first felt like a 'real' vet! I had spayed a deep-chested and considerably overweight cocker spaniel earlier that day. Although at four years of age, Chester had never had puppies, Erika her owner could never quite bring herself to get her spayed. Apparently she had even gone as far as booking the surgery on a few occasions, but never quite been brave enough to allow the increasingly chubby bitch to go through the procedure. I had seen the booking, and half thought she might cancel, but obviously my discussion on the risks of pyometra – a potentially life-threatening uterine infection in older unspayed females – had sunk in.

The surgery was certainly not one of the easiest, as I had to wade my way through folds of fat until I could find the uterine horn and ovary. The uterus already looked thickened and not as healthy as I would have liked, indicating the slow build-up of infection had already begun. Often this sub-clinical infection builds slowly over repeated heats, resulting in an increasingly dull and lethargic animal, which the owner puts down to increasing age. With these dogs, when we spay an older female, the owners report afterwards that the dog has a new lease of life – free from the low grade infection they have been carrying for prolonged periods of time. In Chester's case, I was delighted to be removing the organs before she developed full-blown infection which would make the condition, and the surgery to treat it, potentially life threatening.

Although the surgery was not life threatening, I still sweated as I worked to tie off the vessels along with the ovary, while constantly having my surgical view obscured by rolls of friable fatty tissue. As her surgery was somewhat trickier than operating on a young, healthy, normal-weight dog, I double ligated both ovarian horns and the uterus, suturing the surgical material through the tissue to ensure that the sutures could not slip, which could potentially result in significant post-operative haemorrhage. With each incision to detach the ovary and uterus, I carefully held the stump with the forceps to check that there was no bleeding before releasing it back into the fatty depths of the dog's abdomen. It took multiple layers of sutures to bring the internal muscle and fatty layers together before I sutured the skin, a neat row of sutures hiding the invasive surgery.

I discharged Chester that evening, with strict instructions to keep the Buster collar on at all times to stop her licking at the wound; to keep her quiet until the sutures were removed; and to dramatically reduce her food intake. After the evening surgery, I went home, had dinner and went to bed that night without a further thought. In the earlier days, I would have been worrying about her and would not have relaxed until the three day wound check by which stage further complications were unlikely.

When the phone rang shortly after midnight, it took me a few seconds to recognise the panicky tone of Erika who told me that Chester was lying in a pool of blood. I tried to ask a few leading questions as most owners can be overly concerned by what can sometimes be just normal amounts of post-operative bleeding, but it quickly became apparent that Erika was not going to rest until I saw Chester. Without wasting any further time I agreed to meet her back at the surgery and as I drove the short distance, I mentally replayed the surgery in my mind and was quite happy that my overly cautious nature had ensured that any serious bleeding requiring further surgery to investigate it was unlikely.

Erika struggled to carry the oversized Chester into the surgery and as I went out to help her couldn't help but notice that Chested looked remarkably bright for a dog who had undergone surgery that morning and her tail wagged constantly, clearly enjoying the late-night excursion. I also noticed that the Buster collar which we had fitted her with before she left the surgery was no longer there and that her once-white muzzle was clearly bloodstained. Resting her gently on the consulting table while still wrapped in her blanket, I quickly checked the reassuringly pink gums and her heart rate and pulses, all of which were perfectly normal. Erika, in stark contrast, looked totally blanched and she kept talking anxiously as I tried to listen to the heart rate.

I carefully unwrapped Chester from the blanket to reveal the 'pool of blood', which was little more than a sprinkle from where Chester had overenthusiastically licked at the sutures, resulting in one of the subcutaneous vessels to bleed. Purely to reassure Erika I wrapped a loose, comfortable bandage around Chester's tummy and reissued instruction to her to replace the Buster collar as soon as she got home.

I was almost home before it dawned on me that I was almost as relaxed as Chester about the whole thing. When I had first qualified, even the surgery would have stressed me so much, never mind the phone call to say the dog was lying in a pool of blood. But suddenly, out of the blue, I had felt confident throughout the whole situation and for the first time since qualifying I actually felt like a real vet!

Of course the 'feeling like a real vet' came and went, dealing with different cases and in different situations, but over the years, and although I never did achieve my six-year-old idealist view of becoming the perfect vet, I began to feel less of a fraud.

🐾 🐾 🐾

But more than anything, the things that brought my back to the passage of time were my patients. The tiny puppies that had first presented for vaccinations when I first set up practice on my own quickly grew and became young adults and then with a speed that was at times just too quick, became old. New pups arrived to replace older dogs and it just seemed that the generation went by so quickly as I watched the patients grow alongside my own family. Sometimes old pets were put to sleep and I never saw the owners again. More commonly, in time they would make that difficult first visit with a new pet. Mixed emotions as we all remember the older pet.

I have a terrible habit of remembering people only by their pets so I might meet a middle aged man in the supermarket and without thinking call him Cuddles after the family pet. One lady was delighted when I bumped into her in a local petrol station and called her Angel, after her long-legged willowy lurcher! It was strange that when pets passed away and new pets came, I still seemed to remember the owners by the original pet.

The cycle of life in animals seemed in a way to speed up my own perception of passing time. One day I was received a call from a well-known client, Aoife, to make the final visit for her beloved Sammy. I had known Sammy for a long time – in fact longer than even the owner, as I personally had delivered him many years previously by caesarean section – one of the first caesareans to be carried out when we moved to our new building. Sammy's mother Bella was a Samoyed – hence the name. The father was of questionable origin, as until the day of Sammy and his siblings' arrival, Bella's owner had no idea that she was pregnant. To my mind, Sammy was always 'Kermit', although I never explained why to the owner.

Sammy was delivered late one evening, as is always the case, long past usual clinic hours. By that stage, Molly, now well tall enough to see over the operating table, was an enthusiastic spectator any evening she was free. The first two pups were delivered dead, and had been for some time. I sometimes worried about exposing any of the kids to such stark reality, but they always seemed to take it in their stride. Sammy was delivered next and initially the bright green staining on his coat indicating a prolonged and difficult delivery and his lifeless body suggested that he was also in trouble but as I vigorously massaged his tiny body, he took his first breath and gave a little cry. Once his breathing was steady, I handed him to Molly, who was well versed in neonatal care.

What was to become in time a beautiful glossy snow-white coat like his mother's was bright green. 'Eew, said Molly, wrinkling up her little nose, 'he looks just exactly like Kermit!' For some reason Molly had developed a severe aversion to The Muppets from an early age, veering on absolute hysteria every time they came on the television. In fairness she didn't hold it against him and by the time Bella was waking up, Kermit/Sammy and his two sisters that followed after were very much alive and thriving.

The two siblings were rehomed together to a sister in Waterford, and so I never saw them again. Sammy was the last to find a home, but when he came in for his final vaccination, another client saw him and fell in love and a few days later had eventually managed to talk her husband into letting Sammy join their family. Life was good for Sammy and I was always glad to see him coming in over the years. He was a calm type and never really got himself into any sort of trouble until in his later years.

On a vaccination visit I noticed that despite the thick coat, Sammy had lost weight. On questioning, Aoife agreed that he was drinking more frequently and had become slightly incontinent in the house. I booked him for bloods the following week and when the kidney enzymes were sky high, followed it up with an ultrasound examination. The right kidney was enlarged and had a very obvious growth on it, while the left one looked small and shrunken. The size of the mass on the kidney and the speed with which Sammy was losing weight suggested that this was an aggressive tumour and unlikely to have any positive outcome even with extensive surgery and follow-up treatment.

I discussed the options with Aoife and her partner that evening when Sammy was going home and they rang the next morning to say that they would rather not put Sammy through any further investigation and treatment. For Sammy I was glad, as I really didn't feel it would prolong his quality or quantity of life. It was only three short weeks later that the inevitable call came. Despite all the palliative treatment we could offer, Sammy was now vomiting and refusing to eat. Knowing that it's coming still doesn't make it an easier decision to make and I knew Aoife.

When I arrived, she was sitting on the floor with Sammy, who looked to have aged by years in the few short weeks since I had seen him. Aoife's friend had come to be with her and once Sammy was sleeping soundly from the sedative injection, she asked if I would mind if she went outside with her friend, as she couldn't bear to watch him take his last breath.

And so, just as I had held Sammy/Kermit as he took his first breath, I sat on the floor with his head on my lap as I injected the overdose of anaesthetic and held him as he released his last breath. Although it was a peaceful passing, and in ways less dramatic than his prolonged and surprise entry into the world, it really affected me. I realised that, although in the years of running a practice I had seen many animals come and go, to the best of my knowledge this was the first time I had been with an animal for their first and last breaths of life.

I couldn't go straight back to the surgery afterwards, but found myself sitting on a quiet spot on the beach, wondering about life. Why the drama? Why the heartache? Why the joy? What really is life all about and what are the experiences we encounter trying to teach us?

Suddenly, I felt like my journey was only beginning.

Read more adventures of an Irish vet,
by Gillian Hick ...

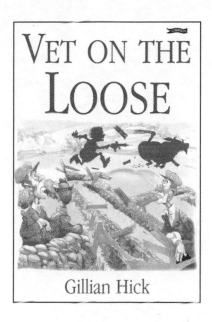

VET ON THE LOOSE

Gillian Hick

Whether castrating horses in Dublin's inner city or dehorning cattle in the wilds of Wicklow, rescuing mangled cats from mongrels or tending to stoned guard dogs, vet Gillian Hick's sense of humour never deserts her in this engaging account of the challenging situations she encounters in the course of her work as a newly qualified veterinary surgeon.

Not only does she have to deal with the animals and their ailments, but she also has to contend with the perils of match-making mothers and macho farmers – not to mention the guys who want to know 'where is the real vet?'

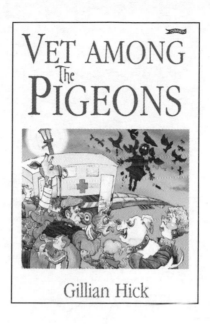

VET AMONG The PIGEONS

Gillian Hick

While based in a mixed animal practice in Wicklow, vet Gillian Hick also travels regularly to inner city Dublin to work in the Blue Cross animal welfare clinic, but finds that sometimes the two lives are hard to combine. From dairy cattle to turkey cocks, from lofty equines to the not so lofty, from six foot snakes to snuffling hedgehogs, Gillian encounters it all as she struggles to improve her own skills and justify her place in the veterinary profession, along with the help of an ever expanding young family of her own.

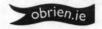